Ultimate Ulcerative Colitis Recipes

A Complete Cookbook of Gut-Friendly Dish Ideas!

BY: Allie Allen

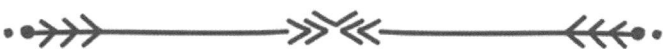

Copyright 2020 Allie Allen

Copyright Notes

This book is written as an informational tool. While the author has taken every precaution to ensure the accuracy of the information provided therein, the reader is warned that they assume all risk when following the content. The author will not be held responsible for any damages that may occur as a result of the readers' actions.

The author does not give permission to reproduce this book in any form, including but not limited to: print, social media posts, electronic copies or photocopies, unless permission is expressly given in writing.

Table of Contents

Introduction 6

1 – Breakfast Blueberry Muffins 8

2 – Golden-Orange Overnight Oats 10

3 – Banana & Peanut Butter Smoothie 12

4 – Egg & Sweet Potato Breakfast Hash 14

5 – Apple & Banana Pancakes 17

6 – Niçoise Lettuce-Free "Salad" 19

7 – Spaghetti Squash Boats 21

8 – Tasty Salmon Burger 24

9 – Chicken Piccata on Pasta 26

10 – Rice Noodles & Tofu 29

11 – Stuffed Eggplant & Pine Nuts 31

12 – Mashed Vegetables 34

13 – Curried Chicken 'n Rice 36

14 – Asparagus & Dressing 39

15 – Chicken & Cheese Pasta Salad 41

16 – Apple & Carrot Soup 44

17 – Peanut & Ginger Zoodles 46

18 – Chicken-Sausage Potato Salad 49

19 – Caesar-Tahini Chicken Pitas 51

20 – Lamb Stew 54

21 – Lentil & Sweet Potato Soup 56

22 – Poached Salmon 59

23 – Scallops & Citrus-Avocado Salsa 61

24 – Roast Tarragon Chicken 64

25 – Butternut Squash & Lemongrass Soup 66

26 – Avocado Chocolate Mousse 68

27 – Pineapple Lemon Cake 70

28 – Almond Butter & Cherry Dessert Bars 72

29 – Fudge-y UC Brownies 74

30 – Banana & Strawberry Frosty Dessert 76

Conclusion 78

About the Author 79

Author's Afterthoughts 81

Introduction

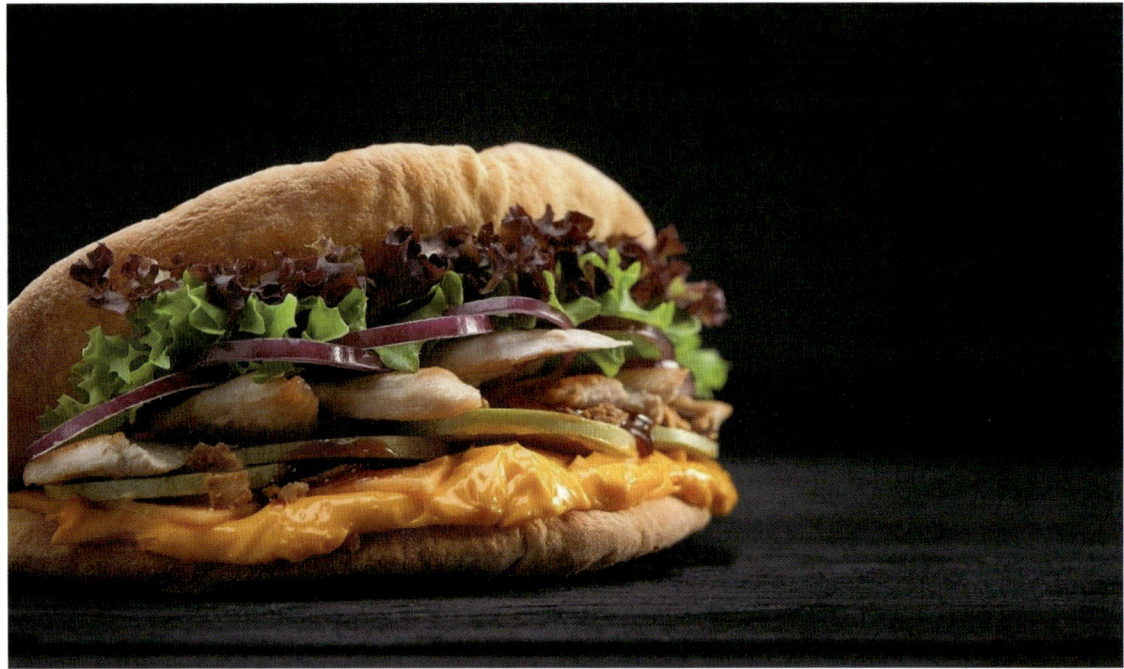

Are you tired of searching for recipes that are gentle on your gastrointestinal tract?

Want some dishes that are no-brainers for most people with UC?

Are you hungry for food that won't make your symptoms worse?

Planning meals doesn't have to be a chore, even if you're living with ulcerative colitis. The dishes in this cookbook will help alleviate abdominal discomfort and other UC symptoms.

The recipes steer clear of the ingredients known to exacerbate UC. Frequent small-sized meals rather than large ones will also help you to deal more easily with your UC.

Tailor the dishes to your own personal UC needs. You may have a worsening reaction to some ingredients that don't affect others.

Despite the potential issues with ingredients, you deserve healthy food since UC can otherwise lead to deficiencies in your nutrition levels. Trial & error will help you nail down the ingredients that work for you and those that don't.

Preparing wholesome meals while you avoid food that might aggravate your UC takes time and patience. But the recipes are free of most ingredients that cause flare-ups. Make some tasty, safe dishes soon!

1 – Breakfast Blueberry Muffins

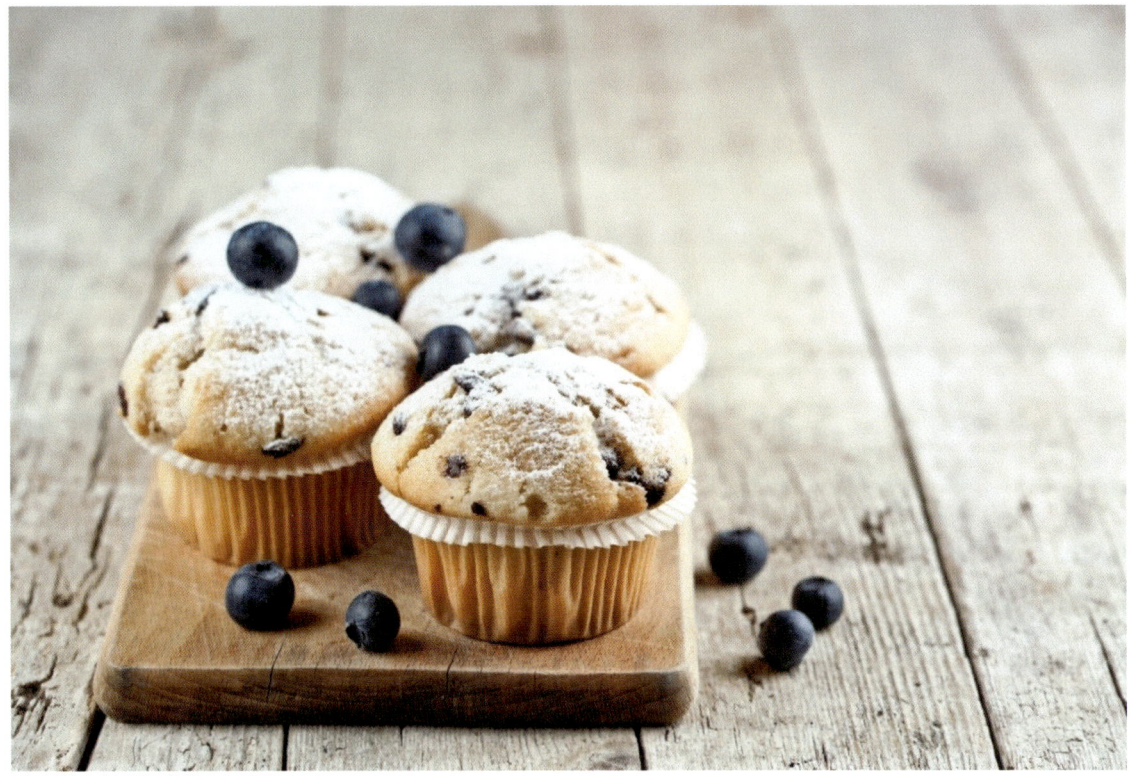

Muffins make a super easy meal in the morning. This recipe uses ingredients that are NOT hard on the stomach, so you can fully enjoy the meal.

Makes 12 Servings

Cooking + Prep Time: 45 minutes

Ingredients:

- 1 & 1/2 cups of flour, white
- 1/2 – 3/4 cup of sugar, white or brown
- A pinch of kosher salt
- 3 tbsp. of melted butter, unsalted
- 2 tbsp. of baking powder
- 1 cup of yogurt or milk
- 1 egg, large
- Optional: 1 tsp. of vanilla extract, pure
- 1 cup of fruit or berries

Instructions:

Preheat oven to 375F. Grease muffin tin cups. Set them aside.

Combine flour, salt, baking powder & sugar in medium bowl. Set it aside.

In separate bowl, mix butter, yogurt or milk, egg & vanilla extract. Pour over dry mixture. Combine together well.

Add fruits. Pour in muffin cups. Bake in 375F oven for 25 minutes. Serve.

2 – Golden-Orange Overnight Oats

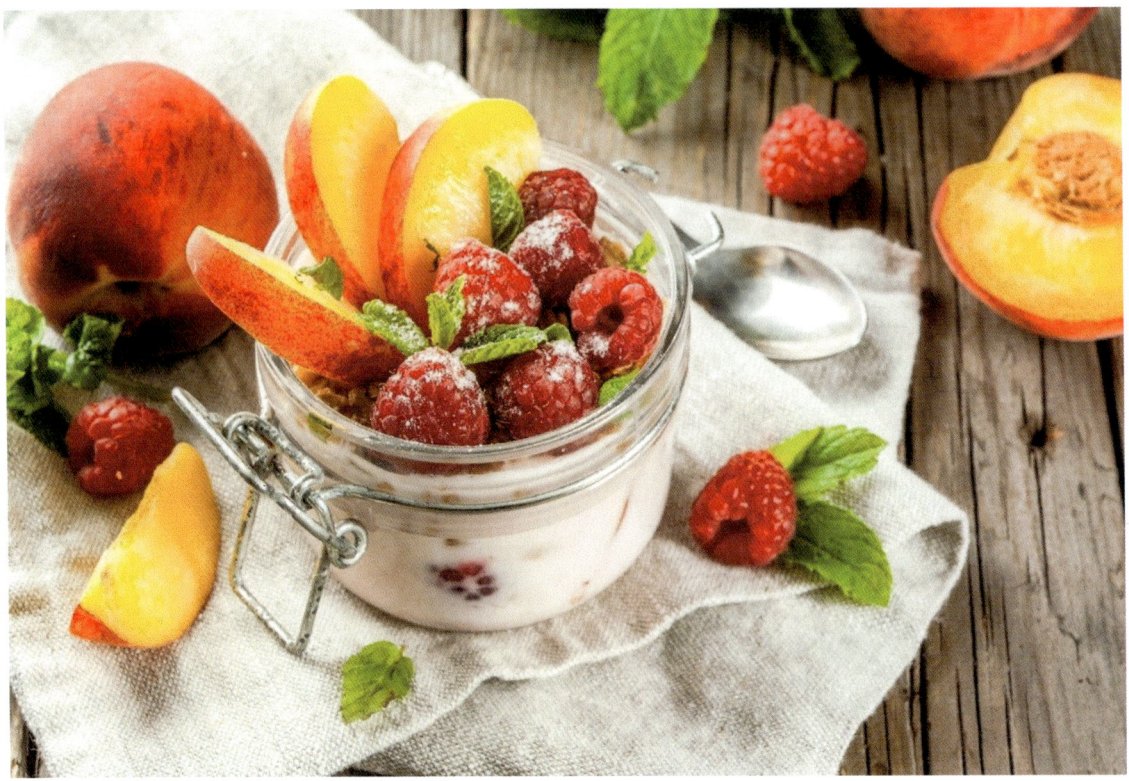

The golden hue of this dish actually comes from turmeric, boosting your levels of anti-inflammatories that are helpful in treating ulcerative colitis. You can top with berries if you want even more healthy, anti-inflammatory compounds in your breakfast.

Makes 2 Servings

Cooking + Prep Time: 10 minutes + 6-8 hours refrigeration time

Ingredients:

- 1 cup of rolled oats, old-fashioned
- 1 & 1/4 cups of soy milk, vanilla, unsweetened
- 2 tbsp. of syrup, maple
- 1 tsp. of orange zest, fresh
- 3/4 tsp. of turmeric, ground
- 1/4 tsp. of cinnamon, ground
- 1/4 tsp. of salt, kosher
- Optional, for topping: berries, fresh

Instructions:

Combine the ingredients except for the berries, if you're using them, in medium bowl. Combine well. Cover.

Place in refrigerator for six hours. You can leave in fridge overnight, if you prefer. Garnish using berries, as desired. Serve.

3 – Banana & Peanut Butter Smoothie

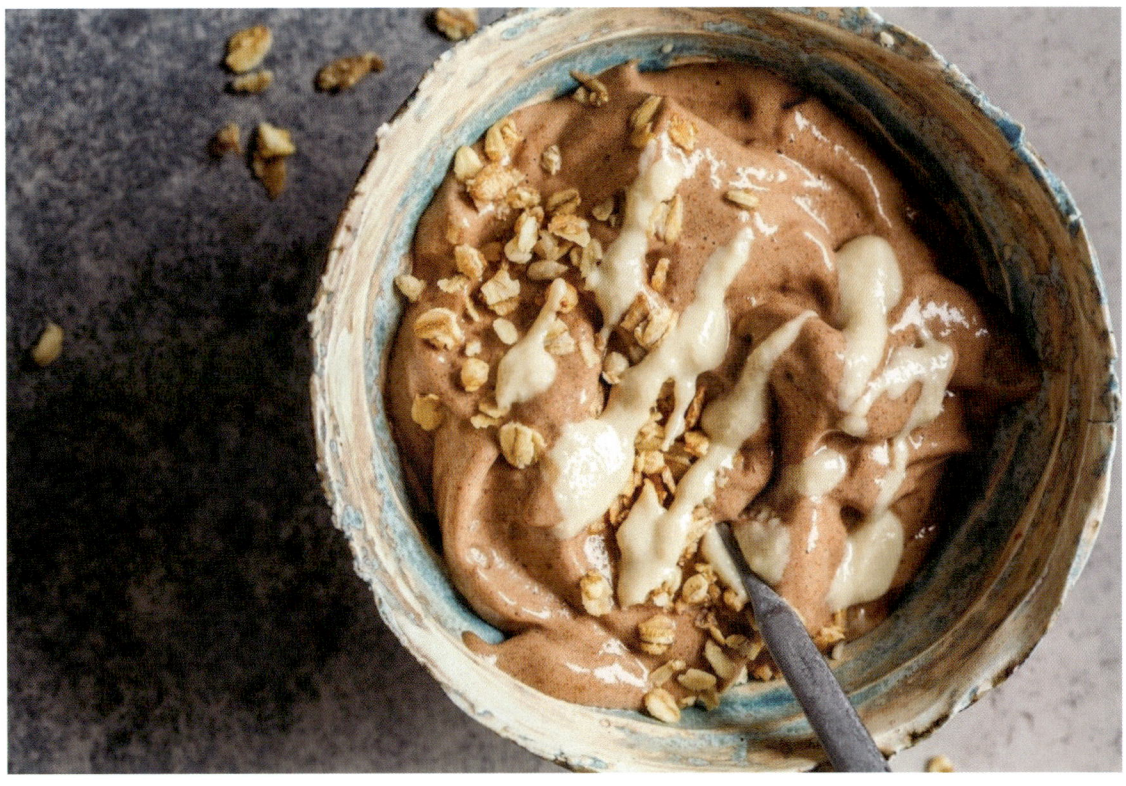

Your body may have difficulty absorbing nutrients if you have ulcerative colitis. This tasty smoothie provides iron and potassium, which your body needs.

Makes 1 Serving

Cooking + Prep Time: 5-7 minutes

Ingredients:

- 1 sliced frozen banana, medium
- 1 cup of spinach, fresh
- 1 cup of soy milk, vanilla, unsweetened
- 1/4 cup of rolled oats, old-fashioned
- 1 tbsp. of peanut butter, natural
- 1/2 tsp. of cinnamon, ground

Instructions:

Combine the ingredients in high-powered food processor.

Blend till fully smooth and serve.

4 – Egg & Sweet Potato Breakfast Hash

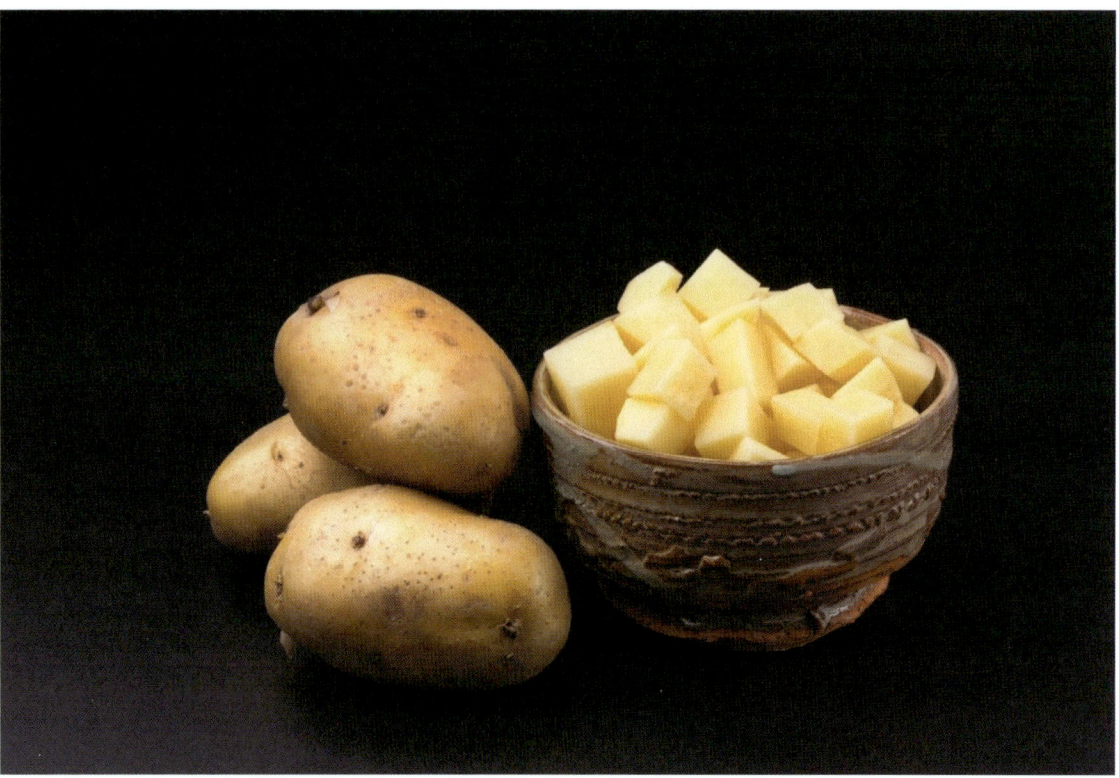

Breakfast hash is an excellent way to increase your intake of veggies. This recipe uses red bell peppers and sweet potatoes for plenty of vitamin A since lots of ulcerative colitis patients lack a healthy vitamin A level.

Makes 2 Servings

Cooking + Prep Time: 1/2 hour

Ingredients:

- 2 & 1/2 tbsp. of oil, olive
- 2 cups of sweet potato, peeled, cubed
- 3/4 cup of chopped bell pepper, red
- 1/4 cup of finely chopped onion, red
- 1/2 tsp. of salt, kosher
- 1/4 tsp. of cumin, ground
- 1/2 tsp. of chili powder
- 2 eggs, large
- 4 tbsp. of salsa, prepared
- 1/2 sliced avocado, ripe
- Optional for garnishing: cilantro, fresh

Instructions:

Heat a tbsp. of oil in large-sized skillet on med. heat. Add the sweet potatoes. Cook till light gold, four to five minutes.

Add 3 tbsp. of water. Cover skillet. Cook till sweet potatoes become tender while occasionally stirring for seven to eight minutes more.

Add a tbsp. of oil, onions and bell peppers to same skillet. Leave uncovered and cook for five minutes or so, till veggies become tender.

Season the hash with 1/4 tsp. of salt, cumin and chili powder. Transfer to two plates.

Add last 1/2 tsp. of oil to skillet. Crack the eggs into it. Cook for three to four minutes, till whites have set. Season with last 1/4 tsp. of kosher salt.

Place an egg atop each plate of hash. Top with avocado slices, cilantro and salsa. Serve.

5 – Apple & Banana Pancakes

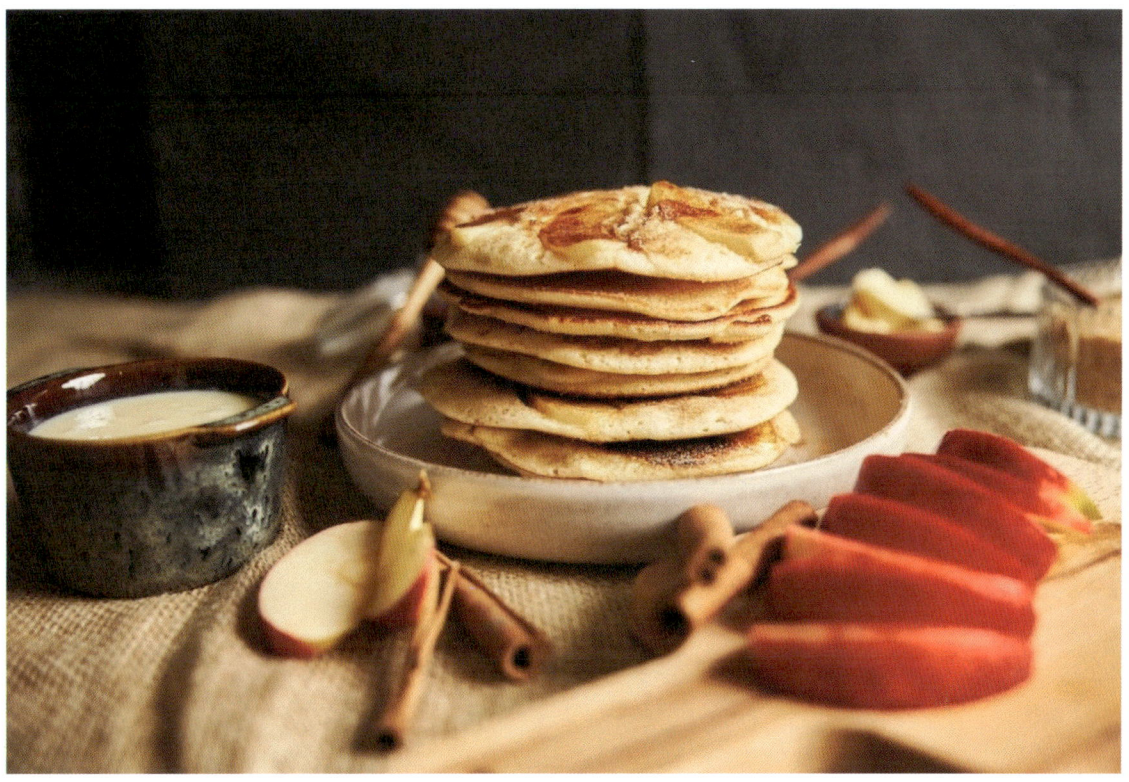

These pancakes offer you the best of both worlds. They're a sweet breakfast treat with no dairy or gluten.

Makes 4 Servings

Cooking + Prep Time: 20 minutes

Ingredients:

- 6 eggs, small
- 3 bananas, ripe
- 1 apple, grated
- 1 tbsp. of oil, coconut
- Optional: honey, pure

Instructions:

Peel bananas. Mash in medium bowl with fork.

Core apple. Grate into banana mixture.

Crack eggs into bowl from step 1. Mix everything together well.

Heat two frying pans. Add a bit of oil into both.

Spoon mixture into pan. Each pan should hold three or four pancakes. Flatten with back of spoon so they're round and thin.

Allow pancakes to cook for one minute, till they become golden brown in color on one side. They should be easy to flip with your spatula. Turn pancakes. Allow to cook till other side is golden brown, too.

Once you have cooked the pancakes, remove them from pans. Cook remainder of mixture till gone. Serve pancakes with honey.

UC Recipes for Lunch, Dinner, Snacks & Appetizers…

6 – Niçoise Lettuce-Free "Salad"

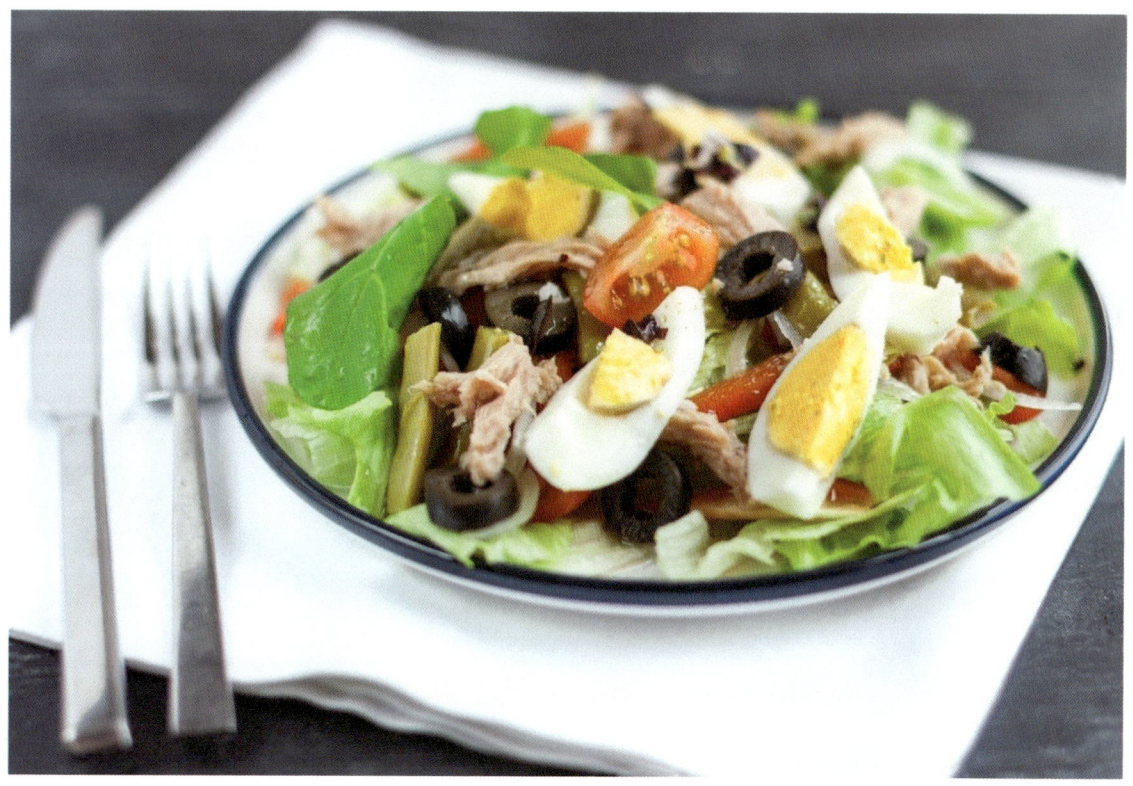

Traditional salads are not usually acceptable fare for people with ulcerative colitis. This "salad" has no lettuce, so you get the flavor without the excess roughage you don't need.

Makes 1-2 Servings

Cooking + Prep Time: 15-20 minutes

Ingredients:

- 2 chopped eggs, hard-boiled
- 1 x 5 or 6-ounce can of drained tuna packed in water
- 1 halved, chopped avocado, ripe
- 12 halved olives, Kalamata
- 3 tbsp. of oil, olive
- Salt, sea, as desired
- Optional: Pepper, black, as desired
- 3 to 4 tsp. of dill, dried

Instructions:

Prepare ingredients as listed above.

Combine the eggs through the olives in large-sized bowl and toss with oil.

Season as desired and serve.

7 – Spaghetti Squash Boats

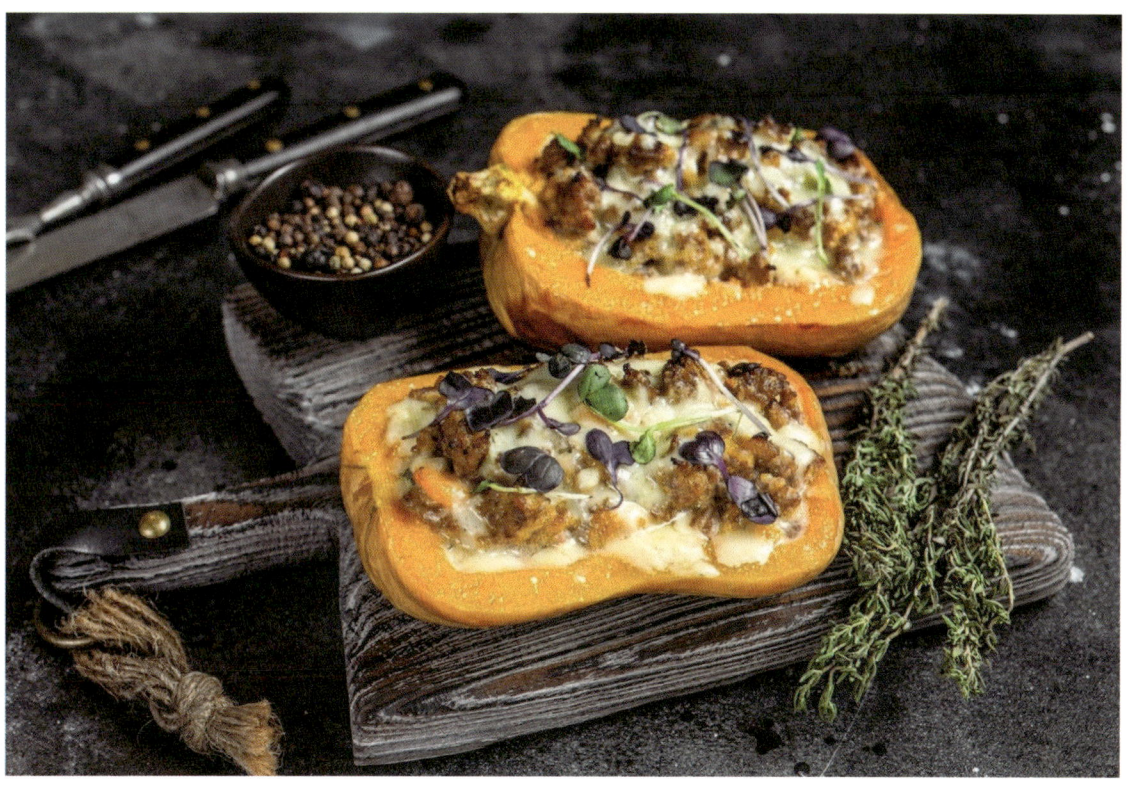

Traditional filled squash boats may include dairy produce and ground beef, which can exacerbate your UC symptoms. Instead, try faux cheese and lean turkey, as this recipe uses.

Makes 4 Servings

Cooking + Prep Time: 55 minutes

Ingredients:

- 2 spaghetti squash, medium
- 2 tbsp. of oil, olive
- 1 pound of turkey breast, ground
- 2 cups of baby spinach, fresh
- 3/4 tsp. of salt, kosher
- 1 x 15-ounce can of tomatoes, crushed
- 4 tbsp. of basil leaves, chopped, fresh
- 3/4 cup of almonds, blanched
- 2 tsp. of lemon juice, fresh
- 1 tsp. of yeast, nutritional
- 1/3 cup of water, warm

Instructions:

Preheat the oven to 400F.

Slice squash lengthwise in halves. Remove & discard seeds. Brush the flesh using 1 tbsp. oil. Place on rimmed cookie sheet with the cut side facing down.

Bake in 400F oven for 35-40 minutes, till flesh becomes fork-tender.

Heat last tbsp. oil in large-sized skillet on med. heat. Add the turkey and break apart while you cook till it is done through, six to seven minutes.

Add spinach and stir. Cook till it wilts, two minutes. Season using 1/2 tsp. of kosher salt.

Add tomatoes and stir. Add 2 tbsp. of basil and stir again. Reduce the heat level to low. Cover skillet and keep mixture warm.

Combine water, yeast, lemon juice, almonds and last 1/4 tsp. of kosher salt in blender and blend till smooth.

Remove the squash from oven. Shred flesh into strands like spaghetti. Evenly fill squash halves with the turkey and vegetable mixture. Top with 2 tbsp. of almond-based ricotta. Evenly garnish with last tbsp. of basil and serve.

8 – Tasty Salmon Burger

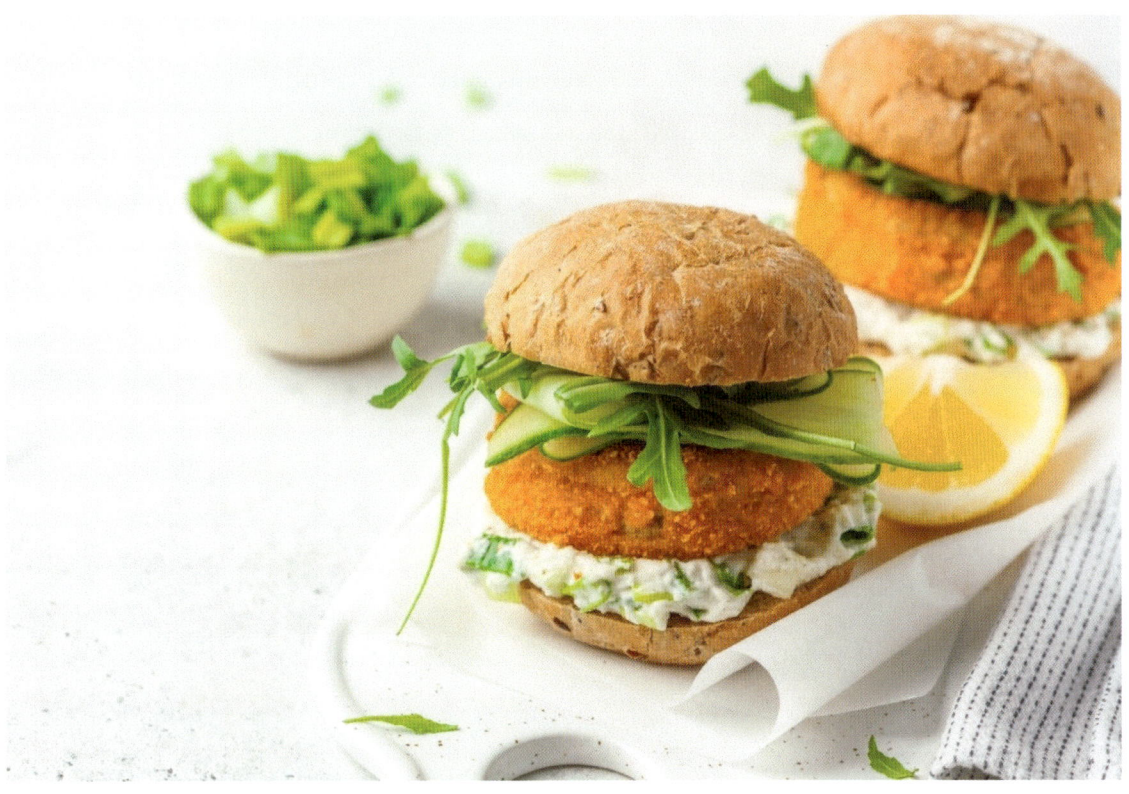

Canned salmon is easy to cook with, and it provides your body with omega-3 fats, which can help in reducing inflammation. You'll love it for lunch or dinner.

Makes 5 Servings

Cooking + Prep Time: 20 minutes

Ingredients:

- 1 egg, large
- 1 x 14 & 3/4-ounce can of salmon
- 1/2 cup of breadcrumbs, gluten-free
- 1 tbsp. of oil, olive

Instructions:

Mix the ingredients together in medium or large bowl.

Shape mixture in five patties.

Add the oil to large skillet on med. heat. Cook salmon patties for a few minutes per side till they have browned. Serve.

9 – Chicken Piccata on Pasta

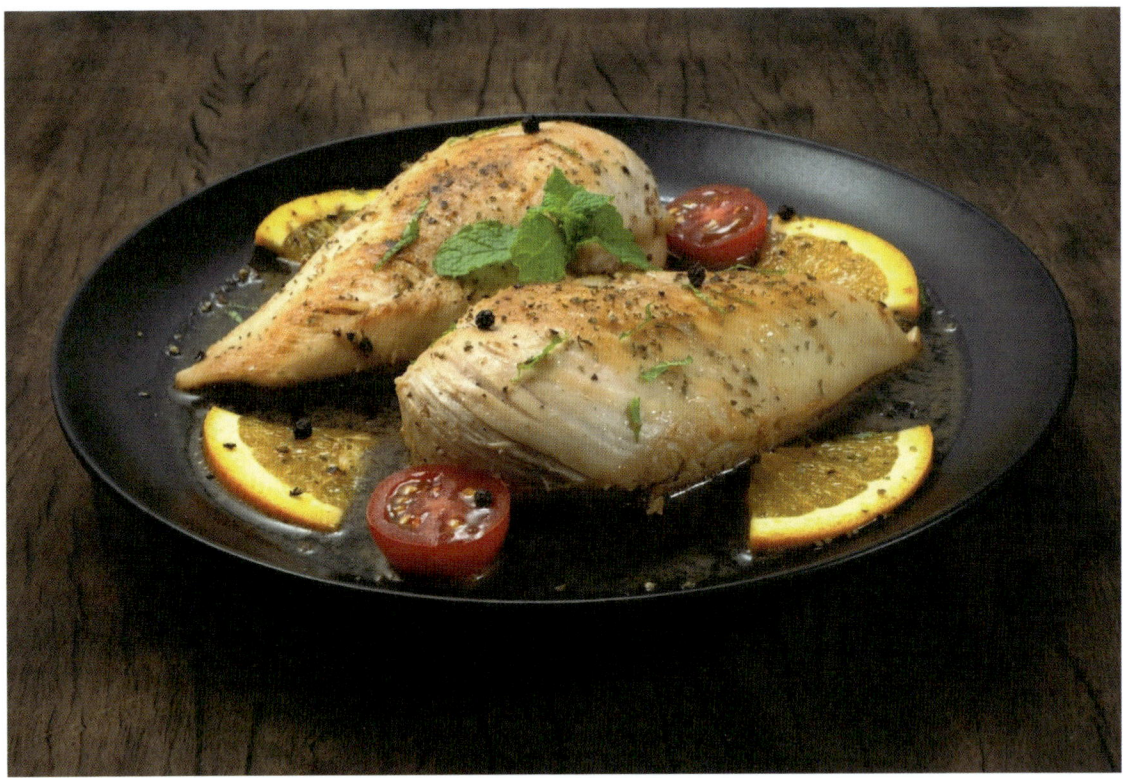

This pasta dish uses less butter, so it doesn't include much saturated fat, which could otherwise be a trigger for your ulcerative colitis. Add a boost of antioxidants by including capers in the dish.

Makes 4 Servings

Cooking + Prep Time: 1/2 hour

Ingredients:

- 10 ounces of pasta, angel hair, dry
- 3 tbsp. of oil, olive
- 3 tbsp. of butter, unsalted
- 1 pound of butterflied, halved chicken breasts, boneless, skinless
- 1/2 tsp. of salt, kosher
- 3/4 tsp. of pepper, black
- 3 tbsp. of flour, all-purpose
- 1 tsp. of minced garlic, fresh
- 1/2 cup of dry wine, white
- 1 cup of chicken broth, low sodium
- 2 tbsp. of lemon juice, fresh
- 1/4 cup of drained capers, brined
- 1/3 cup of chopped parsley, fresh

Instructions:

Cook the pasta using directions on package. Drain. Add to serving platter.

Heat 2 tbsp. butter and oil in large-sized skillet on med-high. Season the chicken as desired. Evenly coat in flour and shake off the excess.

Add the chicken to hot skillet. Cook for three minutes per side without moving it except to turn it, till golden brown in color. Transfer chicken to plate.

Add the garlic to skillet. Stir constantly while cooking for a minute. Then, add the wine and cook for two minutes. Scrape up any brown bits from pan till liquid has been reduced by about half.

Add and stir broth, capers, lemon juice & 1/4 tsp. pepper. Add the chicken back into pan. Simmer for five minutes.

Remove the chicken from skillet. Place atop pasta. Add last tbsp. butter to skillet. Vigorously whisk and combine well.

Pour the sauce over the chicken & pasta. Use fresh parsley to garnish and serve.

10 – Rice Noodles & Tofu

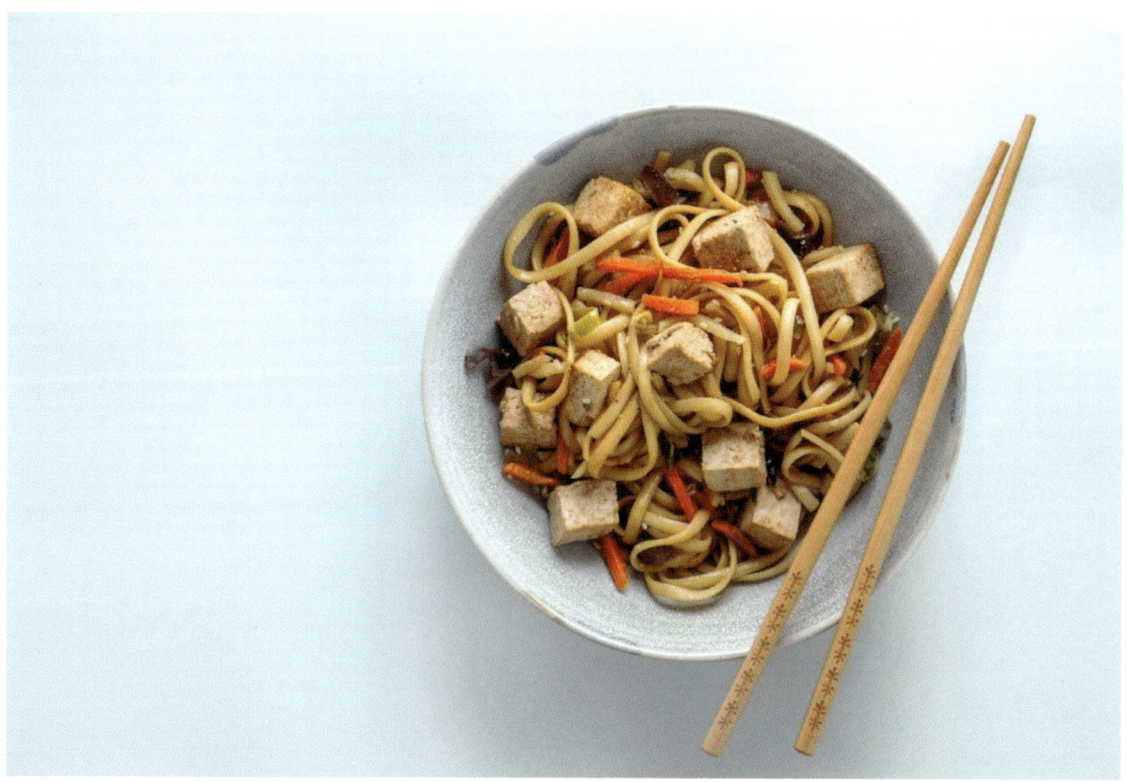

You can lower your inflammation levels by eating a diet that is more plant-based. Using tofu and frozen veggies makes this dish easy to prepare, too.

Makes 2 Servings

Cooking + Prep Time: 55 minutes

Ingredients:

- 1 tbsp. of oil, sesame
- 1 tbsp. of peanut butter, smooth, all-natural
- 1 tbsp. of syrup, maple
- 3 tbsp. of soy sauce, reduced sodium
- 2 tbsp. of lime juice, fresh
- 1 x 8-ounce block of tofu, organic, extra firm
- 2 tsp. of oil, sesame
- 2 cups of vegetables, frozen, like water chestnuts, bell peppers, green beans, carrots, etc.
- Optional: 1 can of corn, rinsed
- 6 ounces of noodles, rice
- Optional: cilantro, fresh

Instructions:

Preheat oven to 400F.

Cut the tofu in small cubes.

Whisk first five ingredients together. Toss with the tofu.

Spread tofu on lined cookie sheet. Bake in 400F oven for 20-25 minutes.

Cook the noodles using directions on package.

Heat 2 tsp. oil in large-sized pan. Sauté veggies till they become tender.

Split the noodles into two bowls. Top with the vegetables and tofu. Add cilantro and serve.

11 – Stuffed Eggplant & Pine Nuts

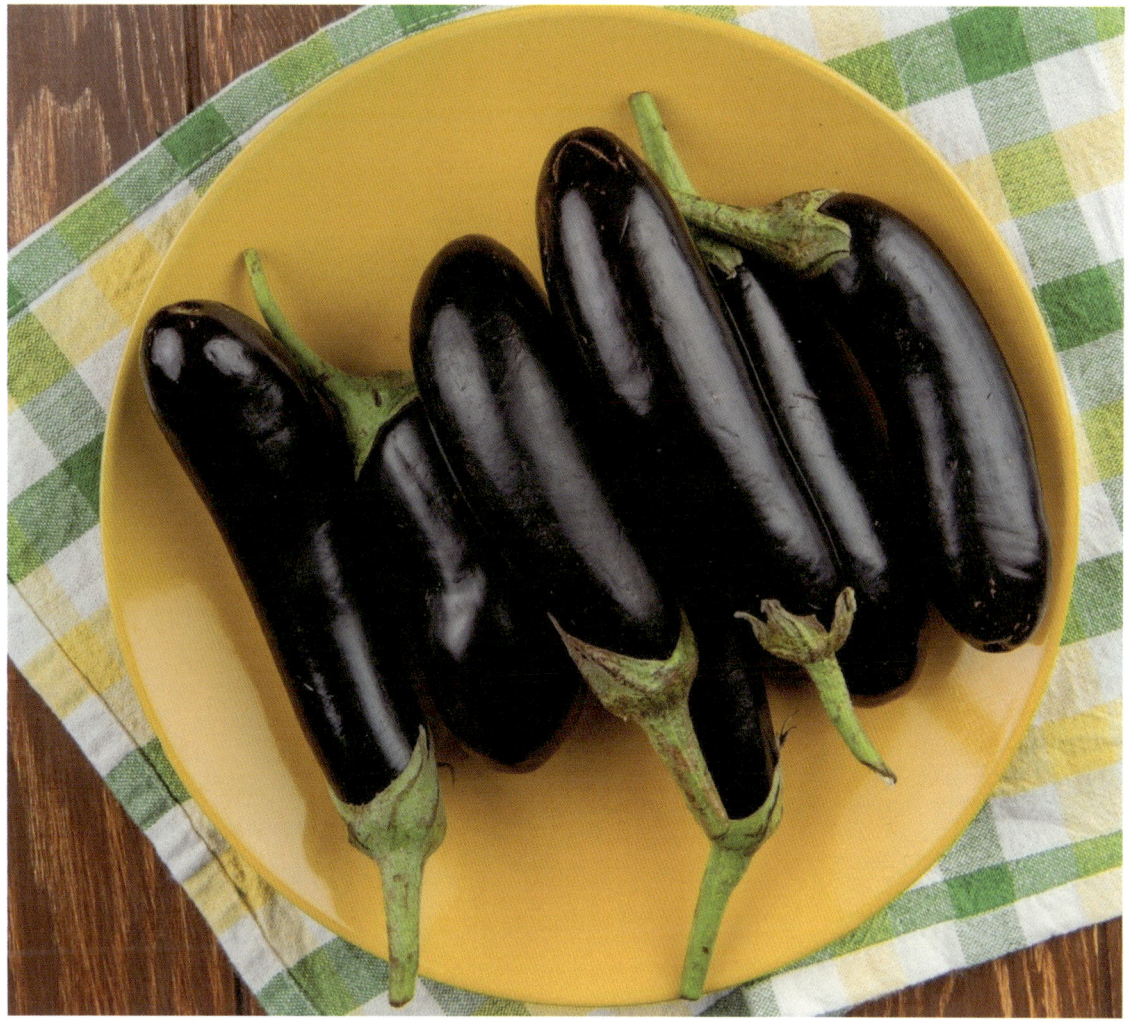

Your ulcerative colitis probably makes you lactose-sensitive, so this recipe utilizes pine nuts & yeast to create "Parmesan cheese." It's a satisfying lunch or dinner dish.

Makes 4 Servings

Cooking + Prep Time: 1 hour & 10 minutes

Ingredients:

- 2 eggplants, medium
- 3 tbsp. of oil, olive
- 3/4 tsp. of salt, kosher
- 3 minced cloves of garlic
- 2 tbsp. of harissa paste, mild
- 1/2 cup of quinoa, dry
- 1 x 14 & 1/2-ounce can of tomatoes, diced
- 2 cups of vegetable broth, low sodium
- 3 tbsp. of pine nuts, chopped finely – you can sub slivered almonds if you like
- 1 tbsp. of yeast, nutritional
- 1/4 tsp. of garlic powder, pure
- 4 tbsp. of thin-sliced basil leaves, fresh

Instructions:

Preheat the oven to 375F.

Slice eggplants lengthwise in halves, through stem. Carve into flesh around perimeter of halves and scoop out the flesh. Set it aside.

Place halved eggplant on cookie sheet with cut side facing up. Then brush with a tbsp. oil & 1/4 tsp. of kosher salt. Bake in 375F oven for 18-20 minutes, till lightly tender and golden brown.

Heat last 2 tbsp. of oil in large-sized skillet on med. heat. Chop flesh from eggplant. Place in skillet. Cook till flesh softens, six to seven minutes.

Add harissa, quinoa, garlic & 1/4 tsp. of salt. Stir often while cooking for two minutes. Add and stir broth and tomatoes. Bring mixture to boil. Lower heat to gentle simmer. Cook till most liquid has been absorbed and quinoa is cooked, 15-20 minutes.

Remove the halved eggplants from the oven. Evenly fill with the quinoa mixture. Replace in oven for 13-15 minutes.

Combine the pine nuts, garlic powder, yeast and 1/4 tsp. of kosher salt in small-sized bowl. Sprinkle over eggplant halves evenly. Garnish using 1 tbsp. basil each. Serve.

12 – Mashed Vegetables

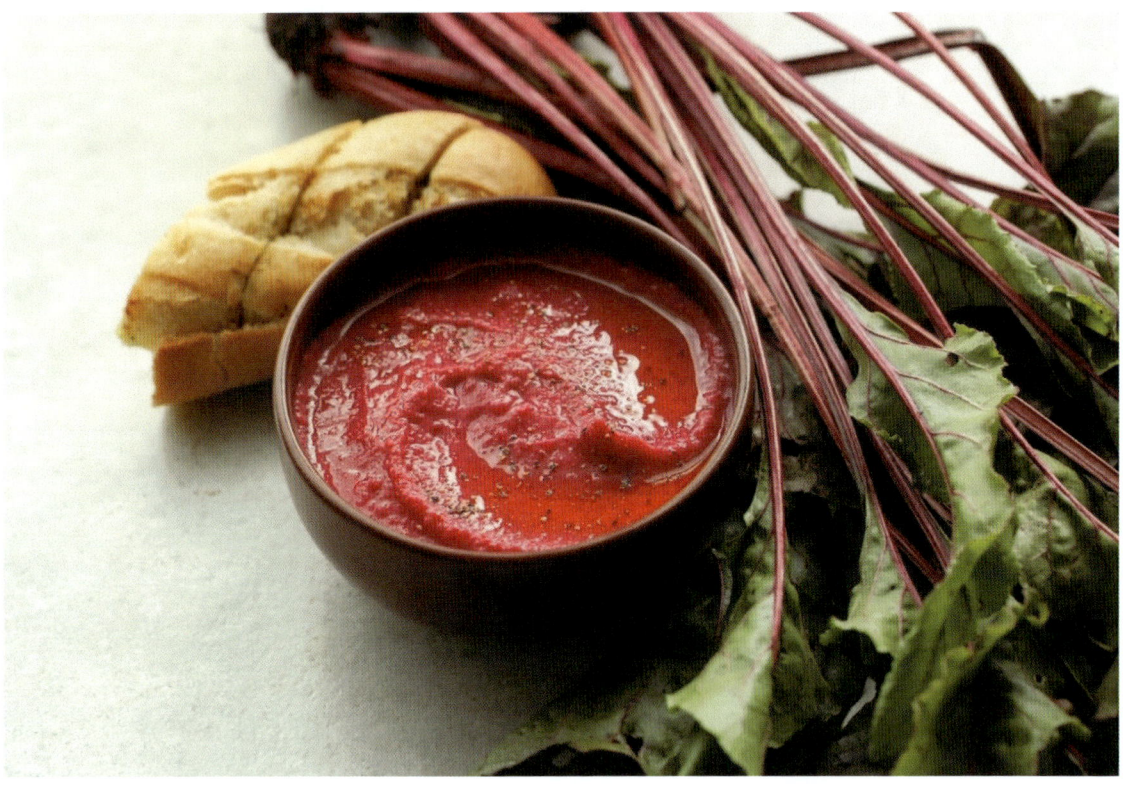

Mashed root vegetables are comfort food and comforting for your gut as well. As long as your veggies are cooked well, they make an excellent choice for people with UC.

Makes 4-5 Servings

Cooking + Prep Time: 15-20 minutes

Ingredients:

- 1/2 cup of stock or broth, low sodium
- 2 lb. of root vegetables like parsnips, carrots, turnips, yams, etc.
- 2 tbsp. of oil, coconut or olive
- 1 tsp. of salt, kosher
- 1/4 tsp. of pepper, black

Instructions:

Steam or boil the vegetables till quite soft and mash them well.

Add the oil, broth, kosher salt & black pepper to the vegetable mixture. Stir well and serve.

13 – Curried Chicken 'n Rice

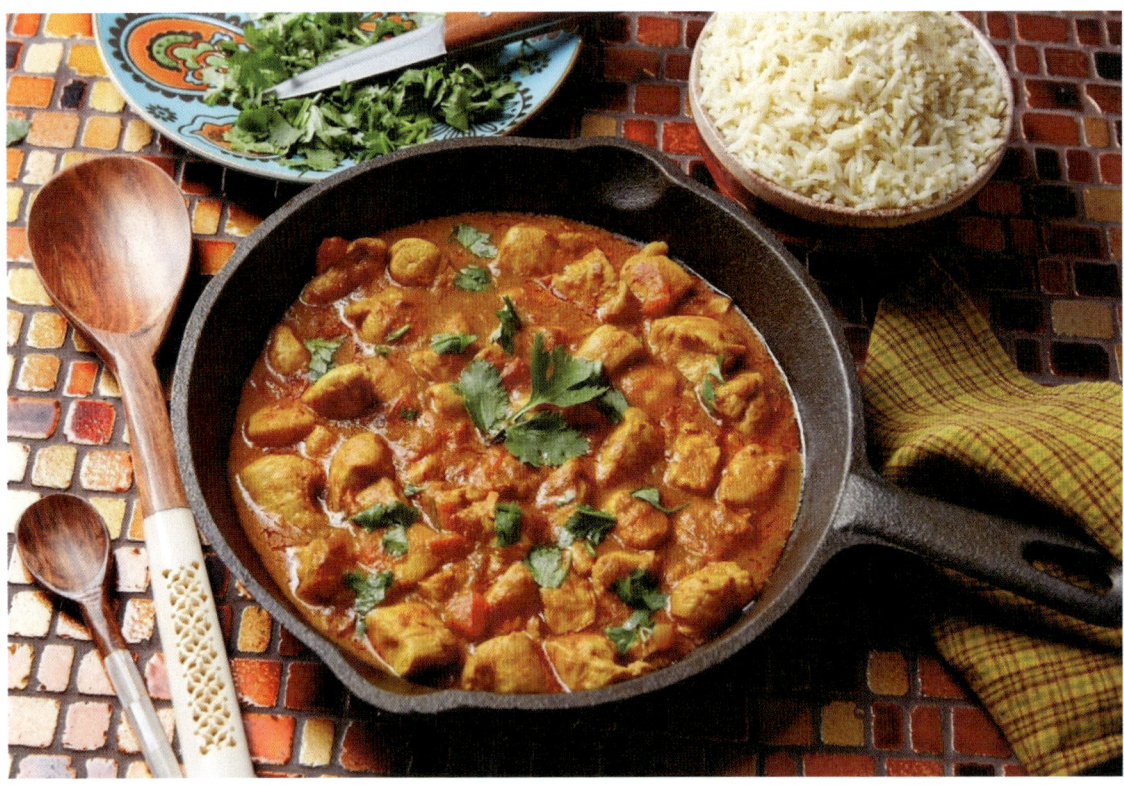

You can actually boost the flavor of a dish by using mild spice blends like the one in this recipe. Shredded meat from chicken breasts is easy on the digestive tract as well.

Makes 6 Servings

Cooking + Prep Time: 45 minutes

Ingredients:

- 2 tbsp. of oil, olive
- 1 tbsp. of curry powder
- 1 tsp. of paprika, ground
- 2 tsp. of ginger, freshly grated
- 2 cups of potatoes, peeled, cubed
- 3 tbsp. of peanut butter, natural
- 2 cups of vegetable broth, low sodium
- 1 x 14 & 1/2-ounce can of tomatoes, diced
- 3/4 tsp. of salt, kosher
- 1/2 tsp. of pepper, ground
- 2 cups of baby spinach, fresh
- 1 & 1/2 cups of rotisserie chicken, shredded
- 1 & 1/2 cups of cashew milk, refrigerated, unsweetened
- To serve: 3 cups of white rice, cooked
- For garnishing: basil, fresh, as desired

Instructions:

Heat the oil in large skillet on med. heat. Add the ginger, curry powder & paprika and cook for two minutes. Stir in the potatoes and occasionally stir for five minutes, till light golden in color.

Add the broth, peanut butter, tomatoes, kosher salt & ground pepper. Bring to boil. Reduce heat level to med-low. Cover skillet and simmer for 18-20 minutes, till potatoes become tender.

Stir in the spinach. Cook for two minutes or so, till it wilts. Add cashew milk and chicken. Stir, combining well. Leave uncovered and simmer for five minutes.

Place 1/2 cup of rice each in six bowls. Top with a cup of curry mixture. Use basil to garnish, as desired. Serve.

14 – Asparagus & Dressing

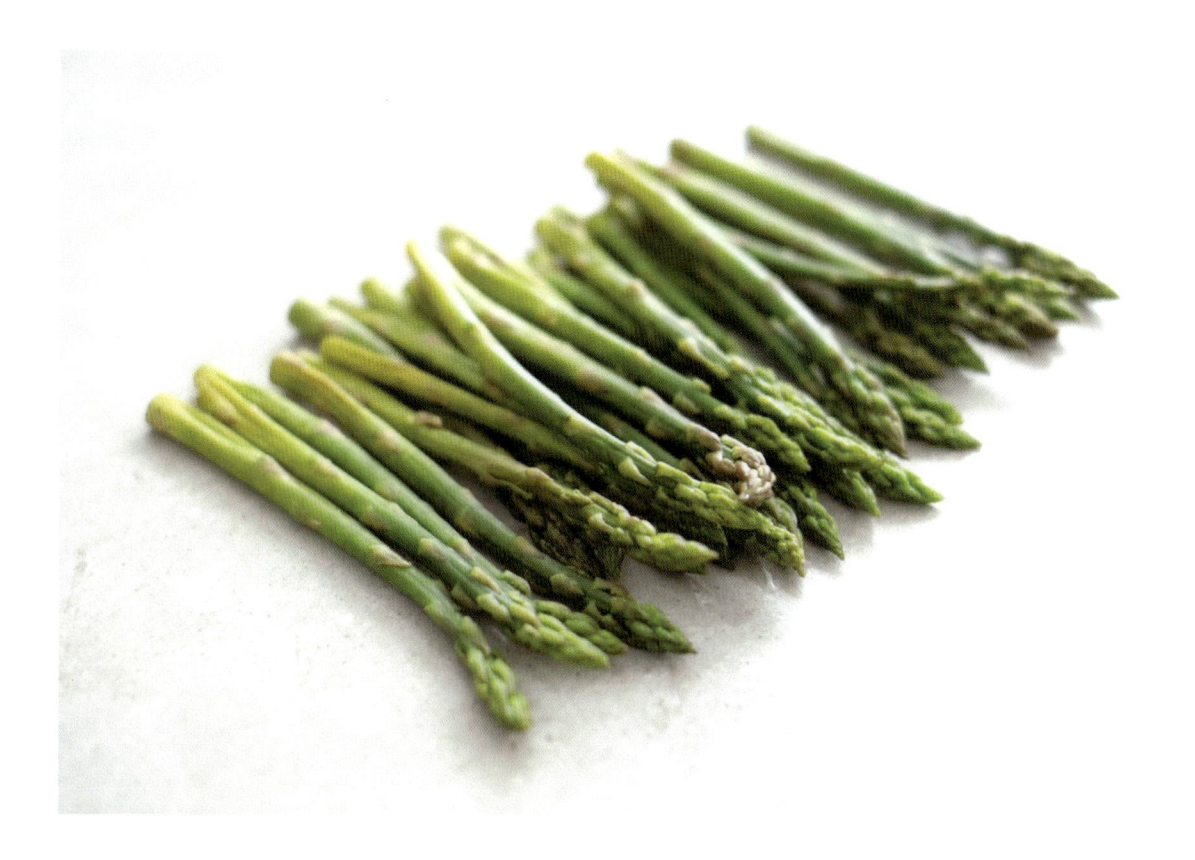

Roasting asparagus mellows its grassy flavor, which highlights this dish. The dressing is made with capers for a unique touch.

Makes 4 Servings

Cooking + Prep Time: 35 minutes

Ingredients:

- 2 bunches of asparagus, fresh
- 1 tbsp. + 2 tsp. of oil, olive
- 1/4 tsp. of salt, kosher
- Optional: 1/2 tsp. of pepper, ground
- 1/4 cup of shallots, chopped
- 1/4 cup of parsley, flat-leaf
- 3 tbsp. of rinsed capers
- Optional: 2 tbsp. of vinegar, white wine

Instructions:

Preheat the oven to 450F.

Trim the tough asparagus ends. Place asparagus on cookie sheet. Drizzle it with 1 tbsp. of oil, plus salt & 1/4 tsp. of pepper, as desired. Toss, coating well. Spread in one layer. Roast and turn once when halfway done, till asparagus starts softening and browning, 12-14 minutes. Transfer to platter.

Place capers, parsley, shallots, vinegar (as desired), the last 2 tsp. of oil & 1/4 tsp. of pepper, as desired, in food processor. Blend till ingredients are chopped coarsely or smooth, as desired. Then top asparagus with dressing and serve.

15 – Chicken & Cheese Pasta Salad

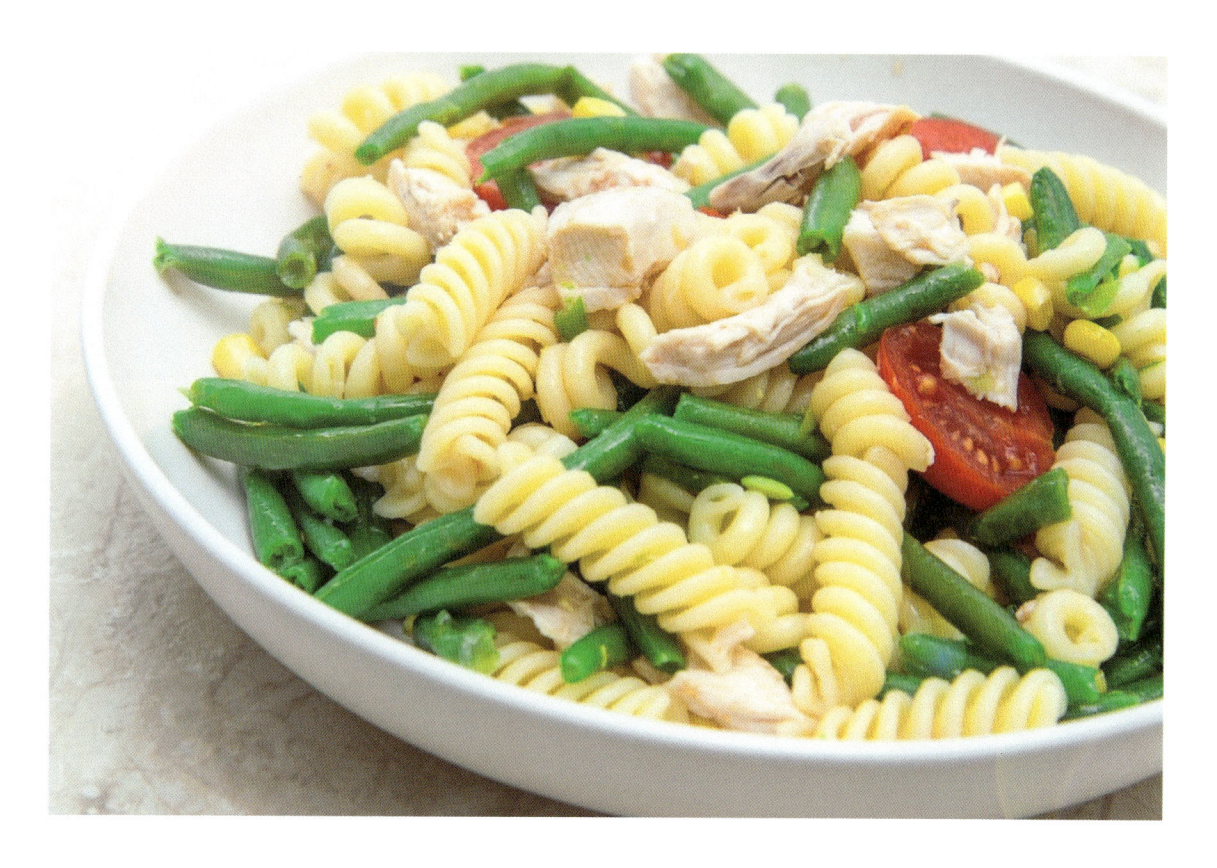

If you have UC and eat a Mediterranean diet, the food fight inflammation and can allow you to have fewer flare-ups. This salad offers a great taste with vegetables and lean protein.

Makes 6 Servings

Cooking + Prep Time: 35 minutes

Ingredients:

- 1 pound of chicken breasts, skinless, boneless
- 1 tsp. of salt, kosher
- 1/2 tsp. of pepper, black
- 1/2 tsp. of paprika, ground
- Non-stick spray
- 12 ounces of pasta, rotini or fusilli, dry
- 2 tsp. of minced garlic, fresh
- 2 tsp. of mustard, Dijon
- 1 tbsp. of chopped oregano, fresh
- 2 tbsp. of vinegar, red wine
- 1/4 cup of oil, olive
- 4 cups of baby spinach, fresh
- 1 pint of halved tomatoes, cherry
- 1 x 14-ounce can of drained artichoke hearts
- 1 x 2 & 1/4-ounce can of drained black olives, sliced
- Optional: 1/2 cup of feta cheese, crumbled

Instructions:

Evenly season the chicken using 1/2 tsp. of salt, pepper & ground paprika.

Heat grill pan on med-high. Coat pan and meat using non-stick spray. Add the chicken. Cook for five minutes per side or till done. Remove the chicken from its pan. Allow to stand for five minutes. Slice in small pieces.

Cook pasta using directions on package. Drain. Rinse using cold water. Place in large-sized bowl.

As pasta is cooking, combine the vinegar, oregano, mustard, garlic and last 1/2 tsp. of salt in medium bowl. Whisk and stir well. Gradually stream in oil while continuously whisking, till combined well.

Add artichokes, tomatoes, spinach and olives in a bowl with the pasta. Toss and combine. Add the chicken, then feta and the dressing. Combine well. Serve.

16 – Apple & Carrot Soup

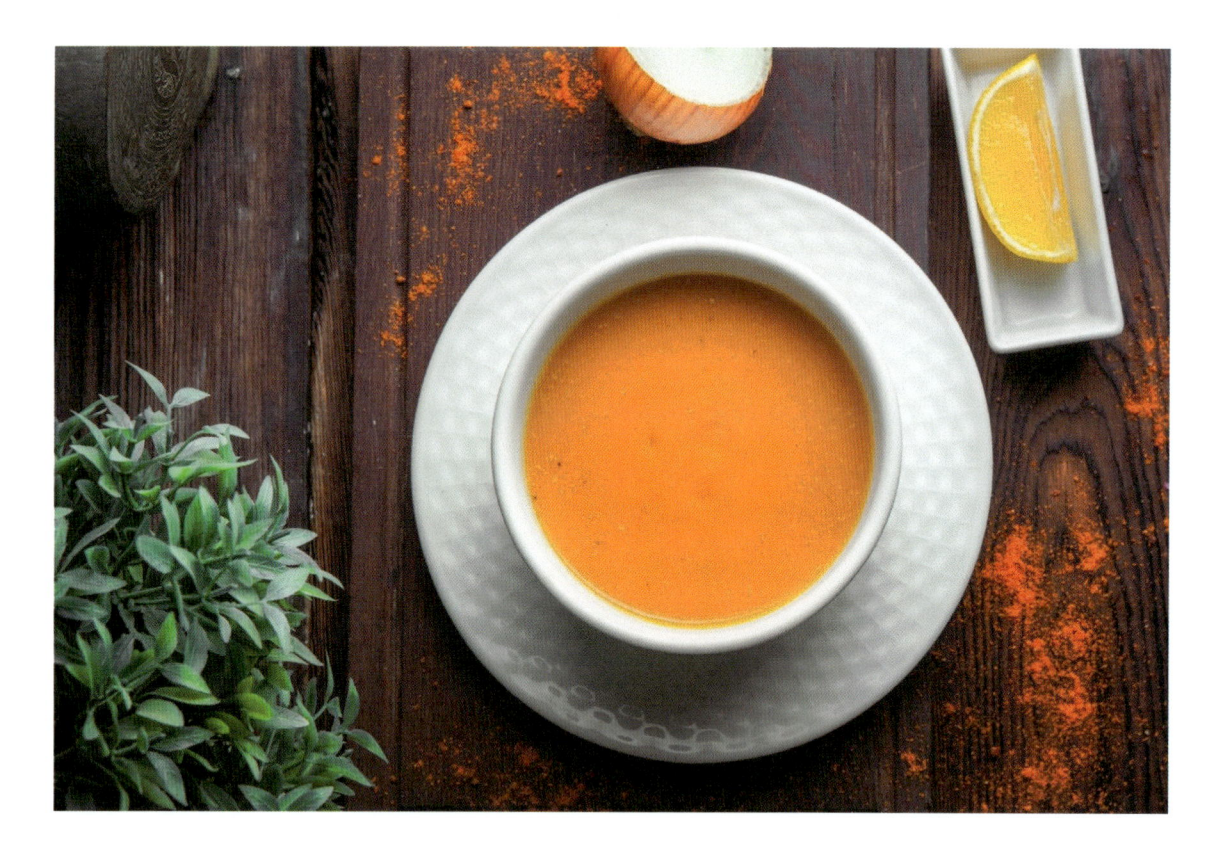

This is a colorful soup that's delicious and simple to make. The best apples to use are McIntosh or any others that will cook up nice and soft.

Makes 8 Servings

Cooking + Prep Time: 1 & 3/4 hours

Ingredients:

- 1 tbsp. of oil, olive
- 1 chopped onion, large
- Optional: 1 chopped celery stalk
- 1 tbsp. of curry or turmeric powder
- 5 peeled, thinly sliced carrots, large
- 2 peeled, coarsely chopped McIntosh apples or other suitable type
- 1 bay leaf, medium
- 4 & 1/2 cups of chicken broth, low sodium
- 1/4 tsp. of salt, kosher
- Optional: pepper, ground, as desired
- Optional for garnishing: 1 tbsp. of chopped basil, parsley or dill

Instructions:

Heat the oil in large pan on med. heat. Add onions & celery and stir. Cook till onion has softened and is translucent, 8 to 12 minutes. Don't allow it to brown.

Add and stir curry or turmeric powder. Add apples, carrots and the bay leaf. Stir thoroughly on med. heat for about two minutes. Add broth and kosher salt.

Bring mixture to low boil. Reduce heat level to low. Cover. Simmer 20 to 25 minutes, till apples and carrots become tender.

Remove bay leaf. Transfer solids to food processor. Add 1/2 cup broth and process into smooth puree. Pour puree back in soup.

Reheat. Season using pepper, as desired. Garnish as desired and serve.

17 – Peanut & Ginger Zoodles

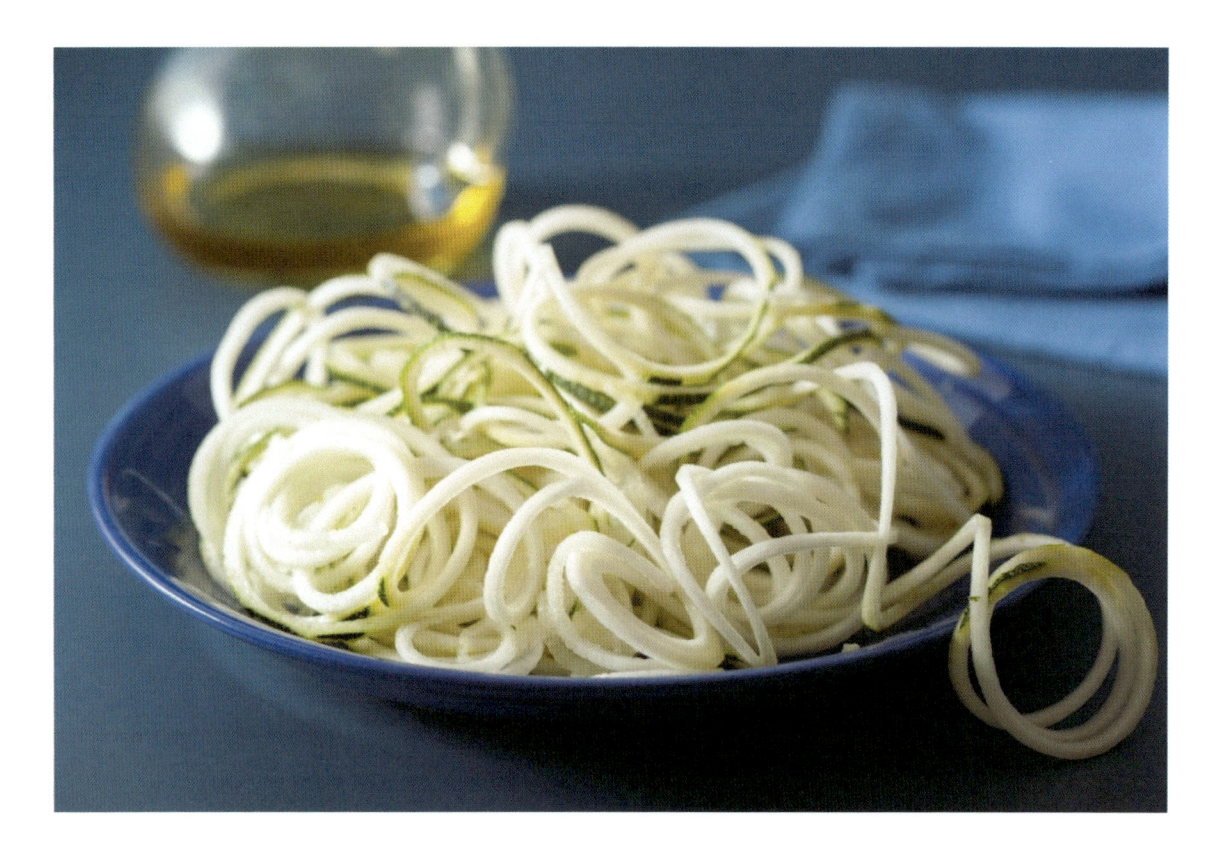

Cooked noodles made from zucchini (also called zoodles) are a good choice as opposed to higher-fiber vegetables when you're experiencing UC flares. The tofu offers calcium, which is helpful for UC patients.

Makes 4 Servings

Cooking + Prep Time: 25 minutes

Ingredients:

- 3 tbsp. of peanut butter, creamy, natural
- 2 tbsp. of soy sauce, reduced sodium
- 1 & 1/2 tsp. of grated ginger, fresh
- 1 fresh lime, juice only
- 2 tsp. of syrup, maple
- 2 tbsp. of oil, olive
- 1 x 14-ounce block of drained, dried, cubed tofu, extra-firm
- 1/2 tsp. of salt, kosher
- 1 & 1/2 cups of carrots, matchstick-cut
- 1 thin sliced bell pepper, red
- 4 trimmed, spiralized zucchinis, medium

Instructions:

In small mixing bowl, combine lime juice, syrup, ginger, soy sauce and peanut butter using a whisk, and set the bowl aside.

Heat a tbsp. of oil in non-stick, large skillet on med. heat. Add the tofu. Cook and stir occasionally till tofu is crisp and golden, 8-10 minutes. Use 1/4 tsp. of salt to season the tofu and transfer it to a medium plate.

Add last 1 tbsp. of oil to skillet. Cook bell peppers and carrots while occasionally stirring for five to six minutes, till they soften. Season with last 1/4 tsp. of salt.

Add zoodles to skillet. Cook while tossing frequently for two to three minutes, so they are heated through, but not yet fully cooked.

Add tofu back to skillet, along with 1/2 peanut sauce prepared above. Toss gently, combining well.

Divide zoodles on four plates. Drizzle last 1/2 of peanut sauce atop them. Serve.

18 – Chicken-Sausage Potato Salad

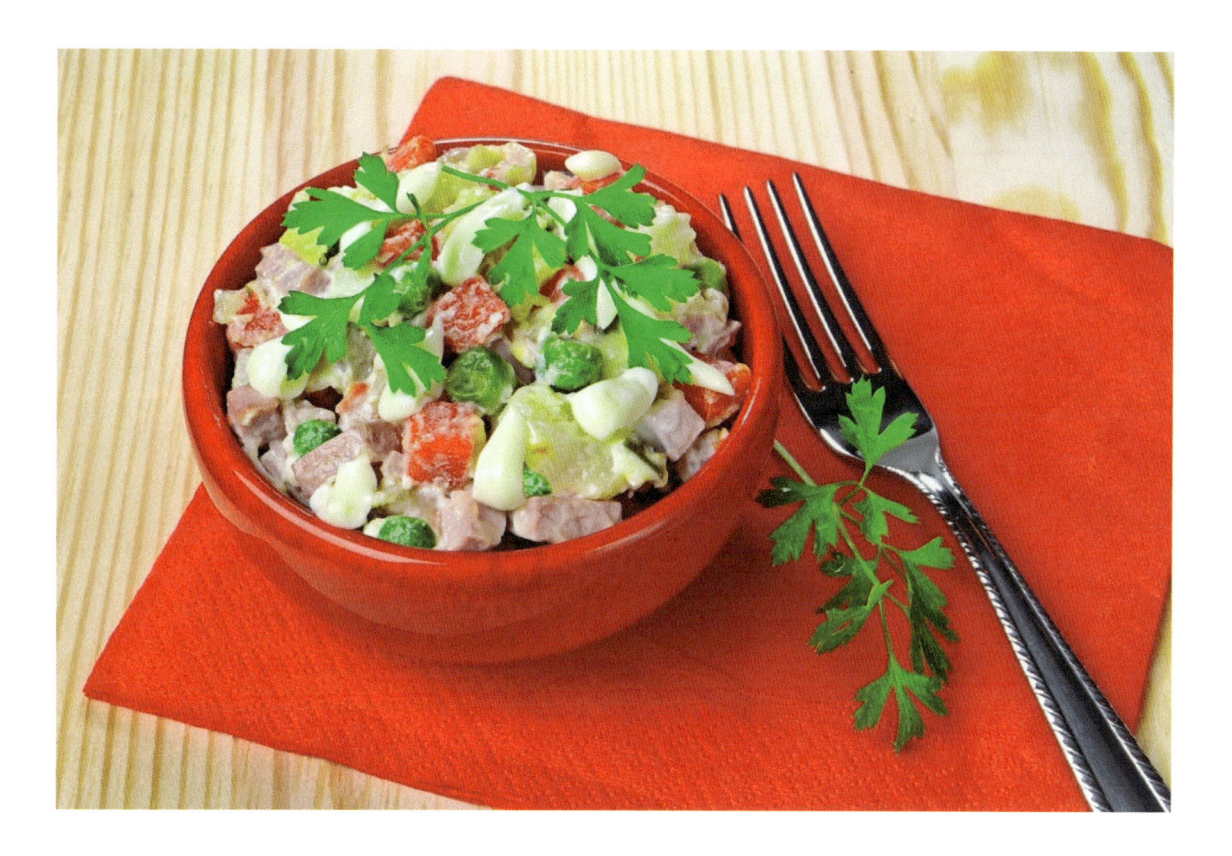

This bistro-style, warm salad is wonderful to share with dinner guests. It has all the feel of comfort food, and its ingredients won't typically cause UC flares.

Makes 6 Servings

Cooking + Prep Time: 55 minutes

Ingredients:

- 1 lb. of halved potatoes, small
- 1 x 5-ounce bag of arugula, packed gently
- 12 ounces of 1/2" crossways-cut chicken sausage, pre-cooked
- Optional: vinegar, cider
- Optional: 1 tbsp. of syrup, maple
- Optional: 1 tbsp. of mustard, Dijon
- 1 tbsp. of oil, olive

Instructions:

Bring an inch of filtered water to boil in Dutch oven. Place the potatoes in medium steamer basket. Cover and steam for 13-15 minutes, till barely cooked through. Transfer potatoes to large-sized bowl. Add the arugula. Use foil to cover and keep potatoes warm.

Cook the chicken sausage in pan on med. heat and stir often for about five minutes, till heated through and browned. Add to the potato and arugula mixture.

Remove pan from heat. Whisk vinegar, syrup and mustard in, if using. Scrape up brown bits, if any. Whisk oil in gradually. Pour dressing over salad. Toss till arugula wilts. Serve.

19 – Caesar-Tahini Chicken Pitas

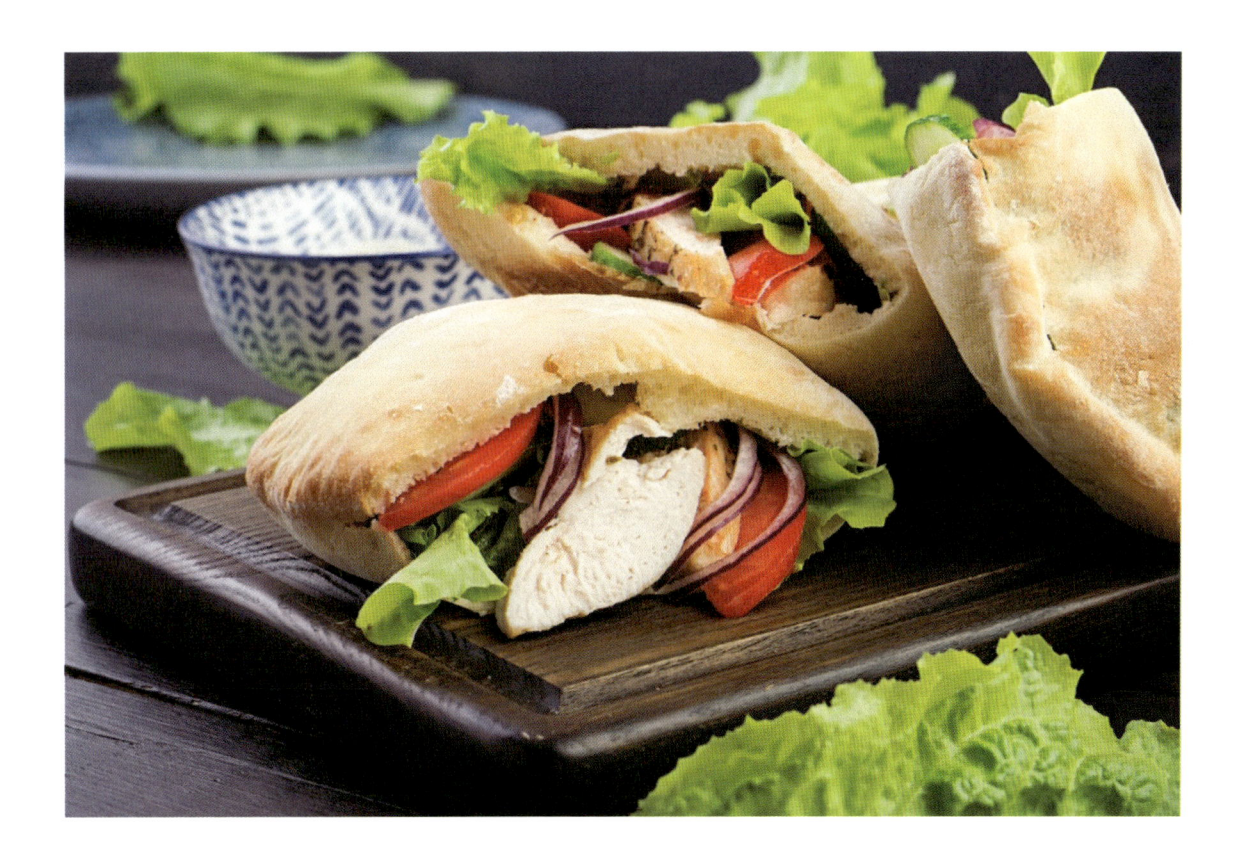

If you're like many patients with UC, you may have an intolerance for dairy products. That's why the dressing here is made with tahini, which is a seed-paste rich in antioxidants. The filled pitas are delicious, too!

Makes 4 Servings

Cooking + Prep Time: 25 minutes

Ingredients:

- 1 pound of chicken breasts, skinless, boneless
- 3/4 tsp. of salt, kosher
- 3/4 tsp. of pepper, black
- 1/2 tsp. of oregano, dried
- 1/2 tsp. of paprika, ground
- Non-stick spray
- 3 tbsp. of tahini paste
- 1 tbsp. of lemon juice, fresh
- 1 tsp. of capers, chopped finely
- 1 tsp. of mustard, Dijon
- 1/2 tsp. of garlic powder
- 1/3 cup of red onion, sliced thinly
- 4 cups of chopped lettuce, romaine
- 1 cup of rinsed, drained chickpeas, canned
- 4 x 3-ounce halved pita pockets, whole-grain

Instructions:

Evenly season the chicken using 1/2 tsp. of kosher salt, pepper, paprika and oregano.

Heat grill pan on med-high. Coat chicken breasts & pan using non-stick spray. Add chicken to pan. Cook for five minutes per side, till done. Remove from the pan. Allow to stand for five minutes. Thinly slice chicken across grain.

Combine the lemon juice, tahini, garlic, mustard and capers. Season as desired. Whisk in 1-3 tbsp. of warm water, till you have a smooth texture.

Combine lettuce, chickpeas and onions in large-sized bowl. Toss with 1/2 tahini dressing.

Evenly divide chicken and lettuce mixture in pita halves and drizzle each using remainder of tahini dressing. Serve.

20 – Lamb Stew

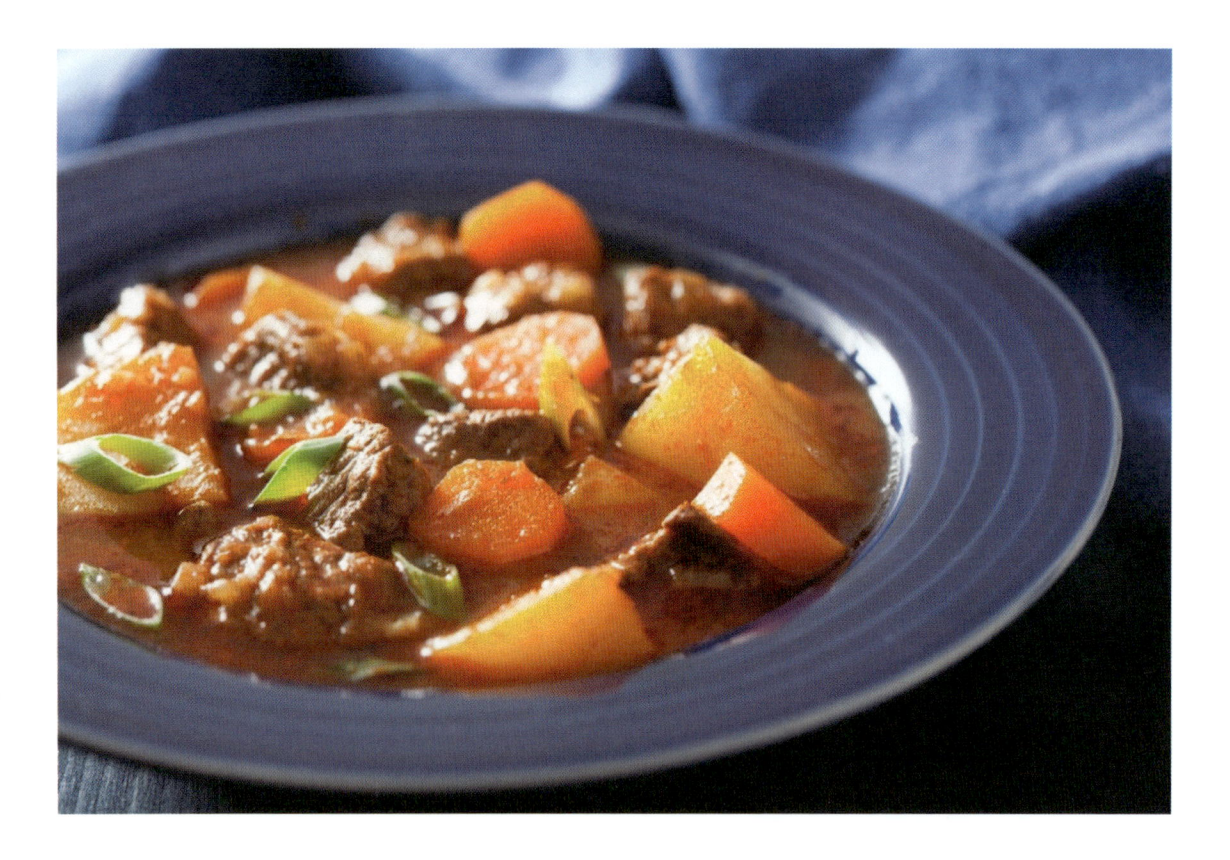

In this stew, you won't brown anything first but rather stew everything together. It's the traditional way to prepare the dish, and it gives you a comfort-food-quality taste.

Makes 8 Servings

Cooking + Prep Time: 1/2 hour + 8 hours slow cooker time

Ingredients:

- 2 lb. of trimmed, 1" cut leg of lamb, boneless
- 1 & 3/4 lb. of peeled, 1" cubed potatoes, white
- 3 halved, washed & thin-sliced leeks, large, only white parts
- 3 peeled, 1" cut carrots, large
- 1 x 14-ounce can of chicken broth, low sodium
- 2 tsp. of fresh thyme, chopped
- 1 tsp. of salt, kosher

Instructions:

Combine the lamb, leeks, potatoes, broth, carrots and thyme in medium slow cooker. Stir and combine well.

Place lid on slow cooker. Then, cook on the low setting for eight hours or so, till lamb becomes tender. Serve.

21 – Lentil & Sweet Potato Soup

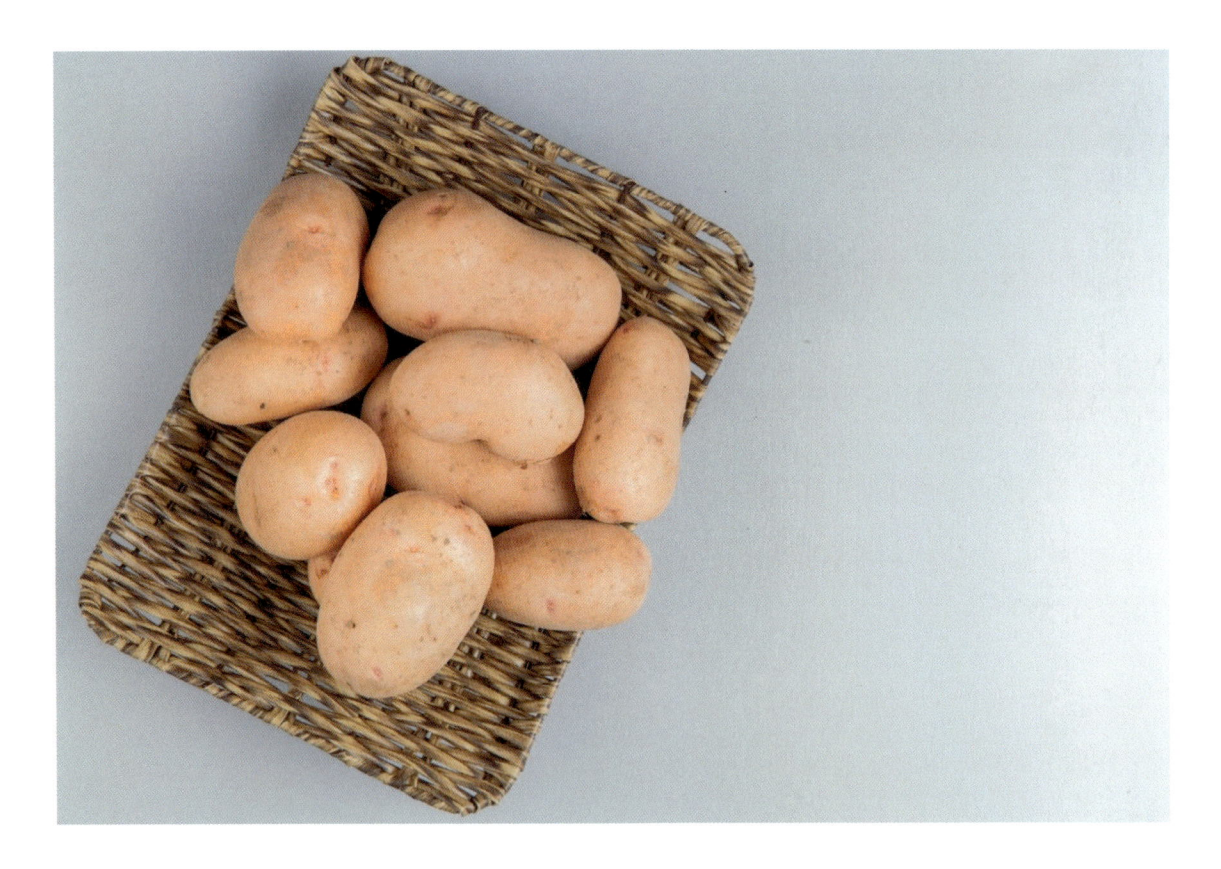

During times of remission, you can enjoy lentils for protein and fiber. The sweet potatoes in this dish add a pleasing taste and beta carotene, too.

Makes 6 Servings

Cooking + Prep Time: 55 minutes

Ingredients:

- 2 tbsp. of oil, olive
- 1 cup of chopped onions, yellow
- 3 cloves of garlic
- 2 tbsp. of tomato paste, no salt added
- 2 tsp. of cumin, ground
- 2 tsp. of garam masala spice blend
- 1 peeled, 1/2" cut sweet potato, large
- 1 cup of uncooked lentils, brown
- 4 cups of vegetable broth, low sodium
- 2 cups of water, filtered
- 1 x 14 & 1/2-ounce can of tomatoes, fire roasted
- 1 tsp. of salt, kosher
- 1 stemmed, chopped bunch of kale, Lacinato
- Optional for garnishing: parsley, fresh

Instructions:

Heat the oil in large pot on med. heat. Add the onions. Cook till they soften, about five minutes.

Add tomato paste, garlic, garam masala and cumin. Cook while occasionally stirring for two minutes. Add the sweet potato pieces. Combine well and cook for five minutes more. Add lentils and stir.

Add water, broth, tomatoes & kosher salt and bring the mixture to boil. Reduce the heat and cover the pot. Simmer for 30-35 minutes, till sweet potatoes are tender and lentils have cooked fully. Add kale and stir. Leave uncovered and cook for about two minutes, till kale has wilted.

Divide the soup in six bowls. Use parsley to garnish, if you like. Serve.

22 – Poached Salmon

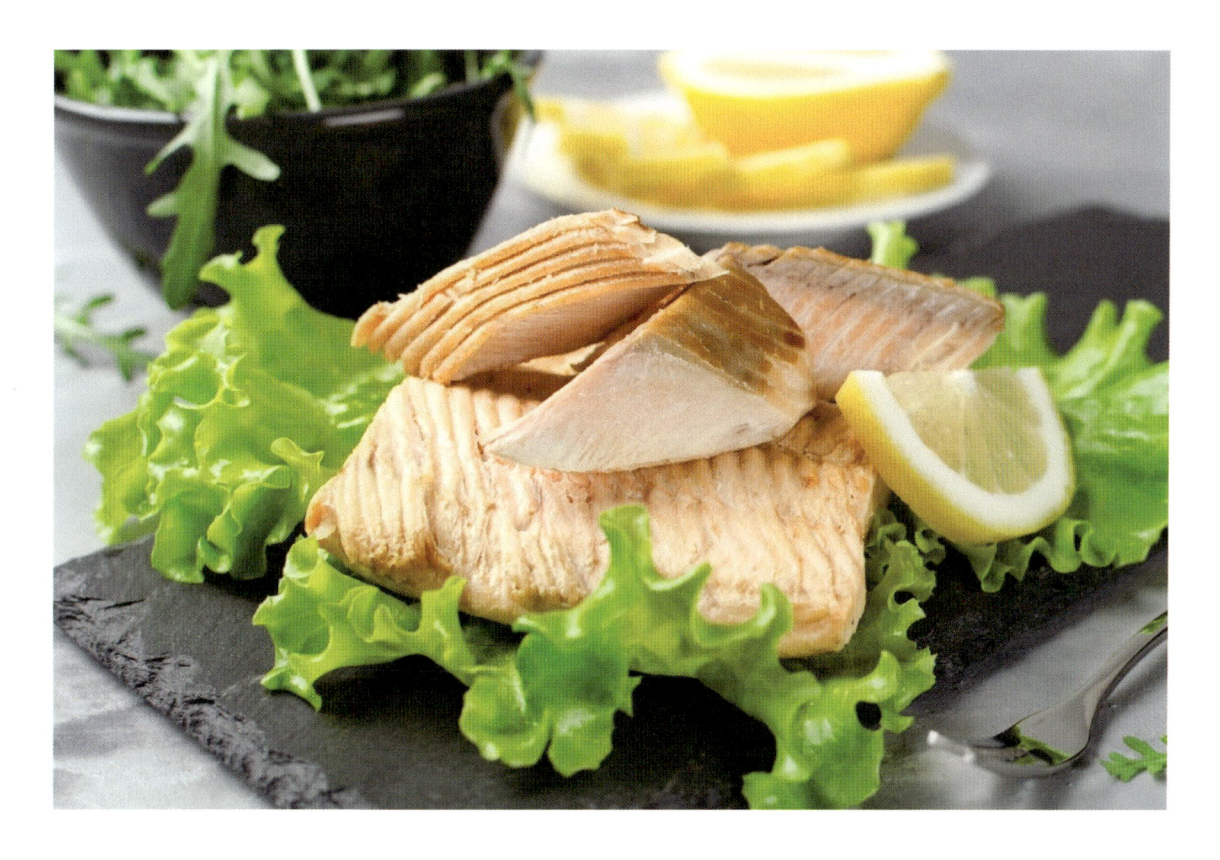

When you bake or poach salmon, you'll achieve moist results and a tasty dish. You can serve this salmon delicacy topped with a favorite sauce.

Makes 4 Servings

Cooking + Prep Time: 3/4 hour

Ingredients:

- 1 lb. of skin removed salmon fillet – slice in four pieces
- 2 tbsp. of white wine, dry
- 1/4 tsp. of salt, kosher
- Optional: pepper, ground, as desired
- 1 medium shallot, chopped finely

Instructions:

Preheat the oven to 425F. Coat 8" baking dish using non-stick spray.

Place the salmon with skin side facing down in baking dish. Sprinkle with the wine. Season as desired and sprinkle shallots over the top.

Cover salmon with aluminum foil. Bake for 15-25 minutes, till salmon center is opaque and salmon starts to flake.

After salmon pieces have finished cooking, transfer them onto plates. Spoon pan liquids over them and serve.

23 – Scallops & Citrus-Avocado Salsa

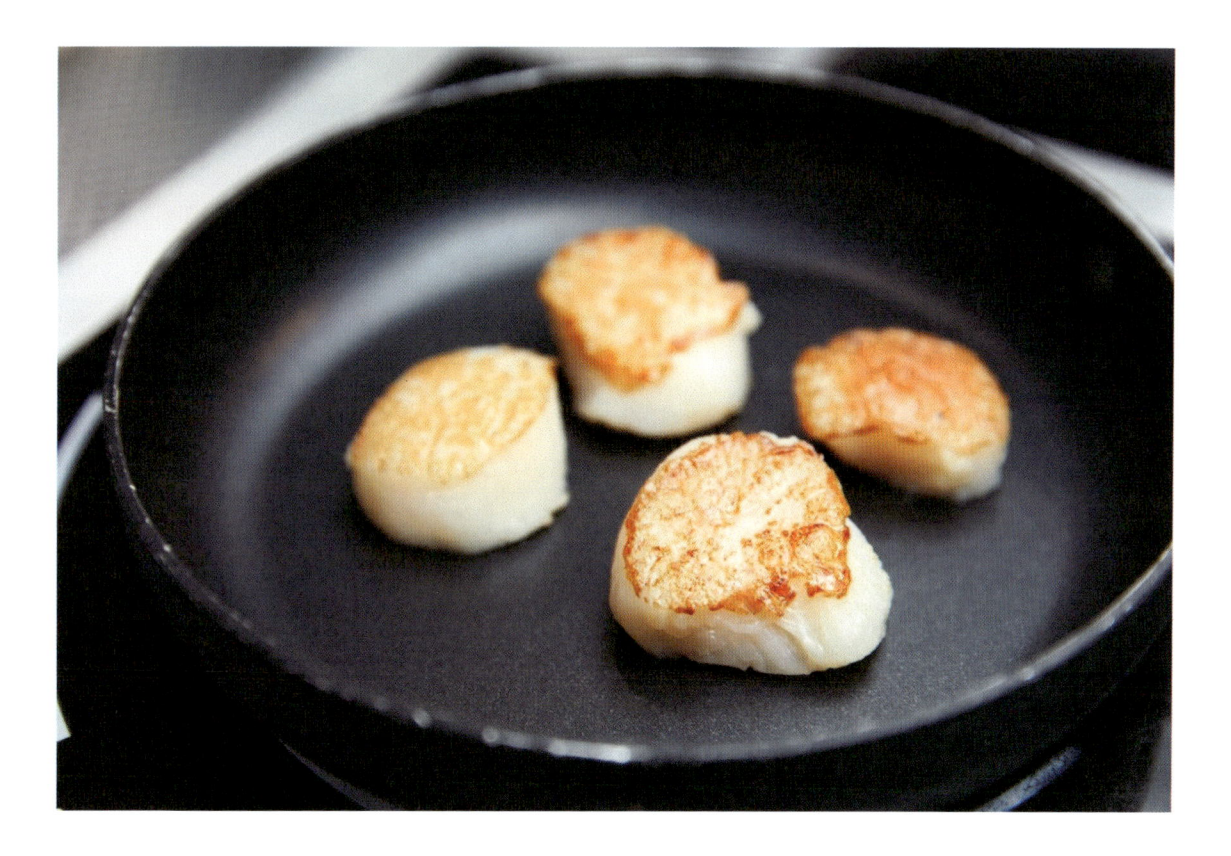

Fruits like oranges have a low roughage level and can be easier on digestion when you're having flares of your UC symptoms. Oranges are actually packed with vitamin C, which helps in enhancing the absorption of iron.

Makes 4 Servings

Cooking + Prep Time: 35 minutes

Ingredients:

- 3/4 cup of rinsed quinoa, dry
- 2 cups of vegetable broth, low sodium
- 2 tbsp. of oil, olive
- 1 pound of patted dry sea scallops
- 3/4 tsp. of salt, kosher
- 1/2 tsp. of pepper, black
- 1 cup of avocado, diced
- 3/4 cup of peeled, diced segments of orange
- 1/4 cup of bell pepper, chopped, red
- 1 tsp. of orange zest, fresh
- 2 tbsp. of orange juice, fresh
- 2 tbsp. of chopped parsley, fresh

Instructions:

Combine the broth and quinoa in small pan. Bring to boil, then reduce the heat level to low. Cover the pan. Cook till quinoa absorbs most broth, 13-15 minutes. Fluff the quinoa and cover it to keep it warm.

Heat 1 tbsp. of oil in skillet on med-high heat. Season scallops as desired and add them to the pan. Cook for two minutes. Turn them and cook two minutes more, till done as you desire. Remove the scallops from the pan. Then, keep them warm.

Combine the orange segments, avocado, orange juice, zest, bell peppers, & last tbsp. of oil in bowl. Season as desired. Toss gently and combine.

Evenly divide the scallops and quinoa onto four plates. Top with citrus-avocado salsa. Use parsley to garnish, as desired. Serve.

24 – Roast Tarragon Chicken

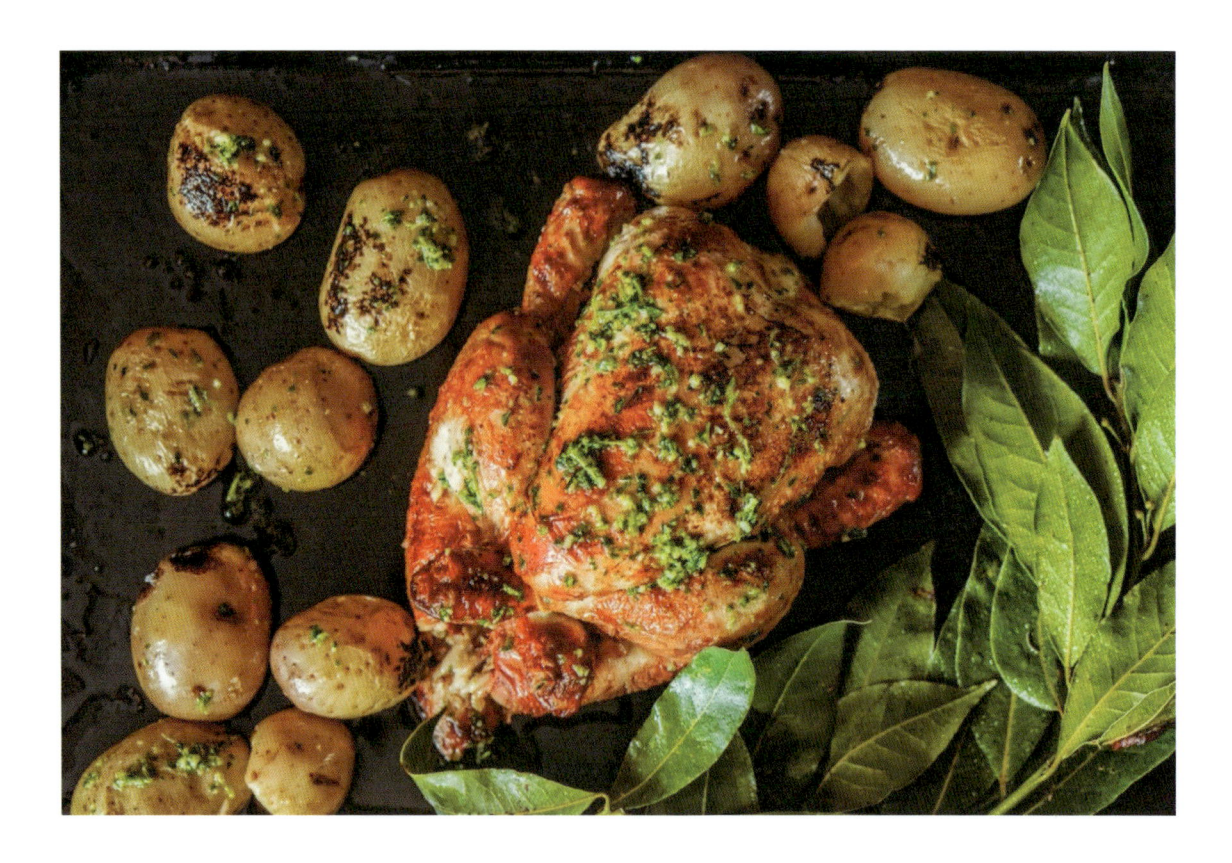

Roast chicken doesn't need to be fussed over or cooked using complicated techniques. In making UC dishes, sometimes simpler is better.

Makes 8 Servings

Cooking + Prep Time: 2 & 3/4 hours

Ingredients:

- 1 peeled, quartered onion, small
- 3 peeled, quartered garlic cloves
- 1/4 tsp. of tarragon, powdered
- 1/4 tsp. of thyme, powdered
- 1 x 5-pound chicken – remove the giblets
- 2 tbsp. of oil, olive
- 1 tsp. of salt, kosher

Instructions:

Preheat the oven to 375F.

Place garlic, onions, thyme and tarragon powders in chicken cavity. Tie legs together using string and close the opening of cavity. Pull wings till tips overlap atop breast and tie them in place.

Rub chicken with the oil and set it in roast pan with breast-side facing down.

Roast chicken for 25 minutes on one side. Turn with breast side facing up. Continue to roast and occasionally baste with juices from pan, till internal temp is 175F, an hour & 15 minutes to an hour & 1/2.

Transfer the chicken to cutting board. Allow to rest for 8-10 minutes. Remove string and carve. Serve.

25 – Butternut Squash & Lemongrass Soup

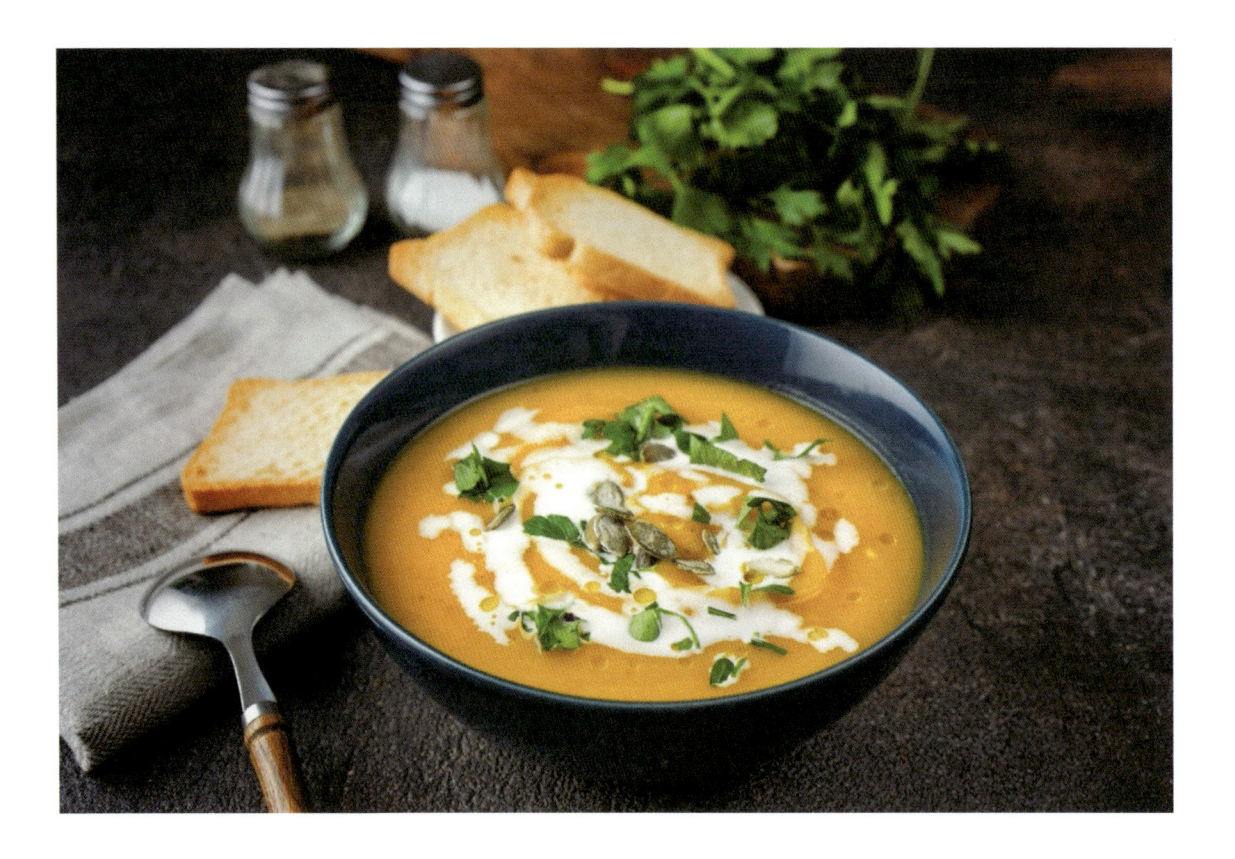

Vegetables that are peeled, blended and cooked are easy on your digestive system when you're experiencing UC flares. This soup is so soothing and also provides anti-inflammatory properties from ginger and turmeric.

Makes 4 Servings

Cooking + Prep Time: 55 minutes

Ingredients:

- 2 tbsp. of oil, olive
- 4 cups of butternut squash, peeled, cubed
- 2 & 1/2 cups of carrots, chopped
- 1 tbsp. of minced ginger, fresh
- 1 tbsp. of lemongrass paste
- 1/2 tsp. of turmeric, ground
- 1/2 tsp. of salt, kosher
- 4 cups of vegetable broth, low sodium
- 1/2 cup + 4 tsp. of yogurt, coconut-milk

Instructions:

Heat the oil in large pot on med. heat. Add carrots and squash. Cook and occasionally stir till light gold, seven to eight minutes.

Add and stir in the lemongrass paste, ginger, turmeric & kosher salt. Cook till aromatic, about two minutes.

Add the broth and raise heat level up to high. Bring the mixture to boil. Reduce the heat level to med-low. Cover. Cook 40-45 minutes till vegetables become quite tender.

Pour the mixture carefully into your blender. Add the half-cup of yogurt. Remove blender lid center piece so steam can escape. Secure the lid. Place clean towel over lid opening and process till smooth.

Evenly divide soup in six bowls. Swirl a tsp. of yogurt in each bowl and serve.

26 – Avocado Chocolate Mousse

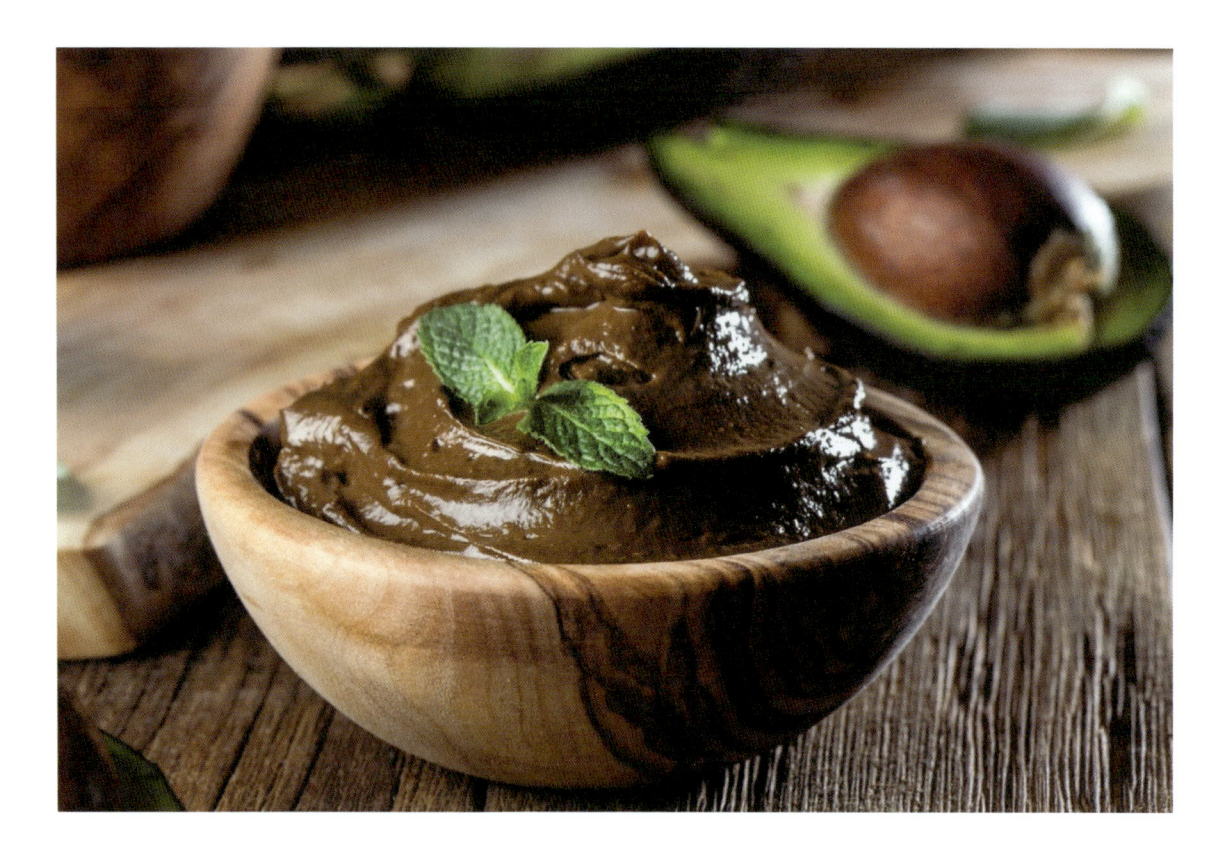

Even if you're experiencing UC flares, you still deserve some desserts. It's a form of caring for yourself, and this dish is a great potassium source, too.

Makes 4 Servings

Cooking + Prep Time: 1 & 1/4 hours

Ingredients:

- 2 large avocados, ripe
- 1/4 cup of cocoa powder, unsweetened
- 2 tbsp. of baking cocoa, dark
- 1/4 cup of syrup, maple
- 3 tbsp. of cashew milk, soy milk or almond milk, unsweetened
- 1 tsp. of vanilla extract, pure
- 1/4 tsp. of salt, sea
- Optional, for garnishing: raspberries, fresh

Instructions:

Place ingredients except raspberries in food processor and blend till smooth.

Transfer to bowl. Chill for an hour. Then, divide into four bowls and top with the raspberries, as desired. Serve.

27 – Pineapple Lemon Cake

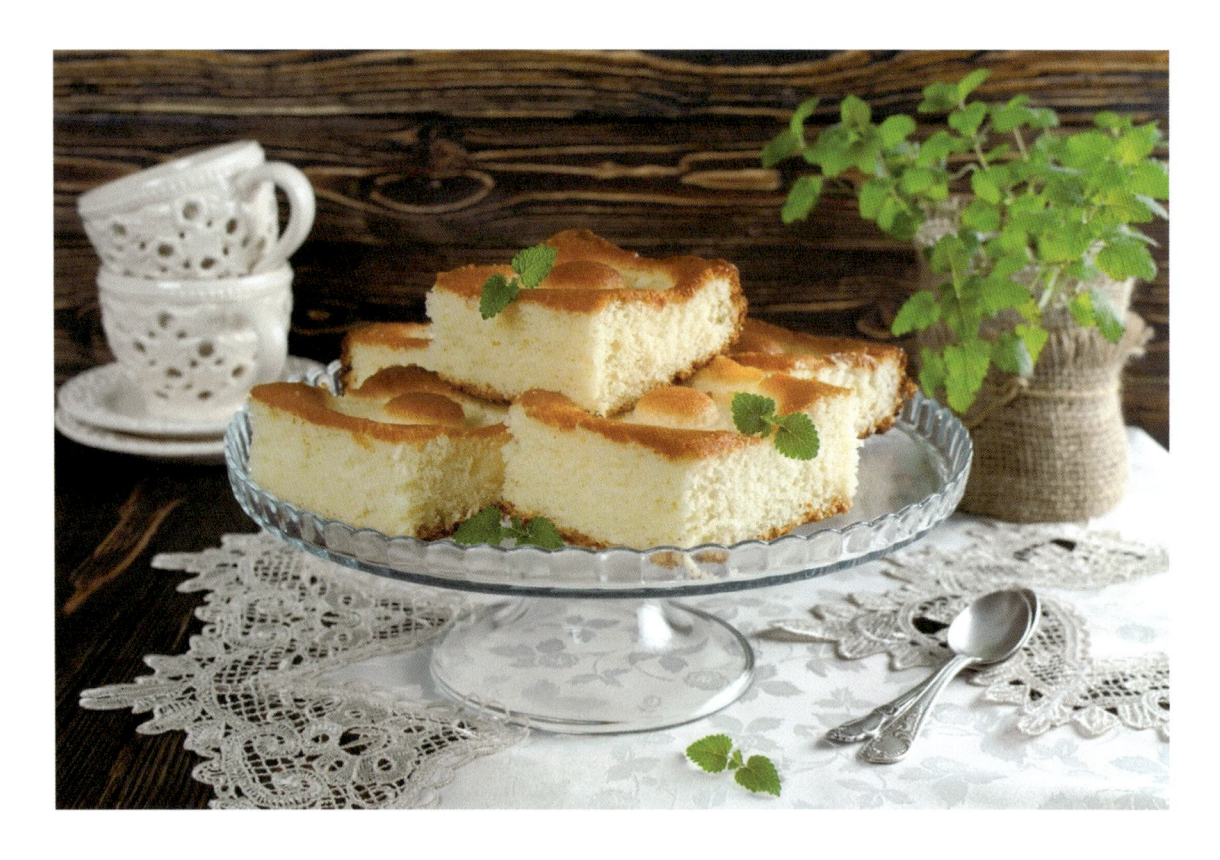

This is a plant-based cake recipe that utilizes maple syrup in lieu of refined sugar. When you flip it over to cool, its sweet juices make their way into the cake itself.

Makes 8 Servings

Cooking + Prep Time: 55 minutes

Ingredients:

- 1 fresh pineapple, cut in chunks or rings
- 1 cup of milk, nut
- 1 & 1/2 cups of flour, gluten free
- 3/4 cup of syrup, maple
- 1 tbsp. of lemon juice, fresh
- 2 & 1/4 tsp. of baking powder
- 1 & 1/2 tsp. of vanilla, pure
- 1/2 tsp. of cinnamon, ground
- 1/4 tsp. of nutmeg, ground

Instructions:

Preheat the oven to 350F.

Drizzle 1/4 cup of lemon and syrup on bottom of 9" non-stick cake pan and cover bottom with chunks or rings of pineapple.

Mix the dry ingredients in small mixing bowl.

In separate bowl, whisk the nut milk, vanilla & 1/2 cup of syrup. Add the dry ingredients. Combine by stirring.

Pour the batter over chunks or rings of pineapple. Bake in 350F oven for 40 minutes. You should be able to insert a toothpick in middle and have it come back clean.

Cool for 8-10 minutes. Flip cake upside down on plate. Cool a bit and serve.

28 – Almond Butter & Cherry Dessert Bars

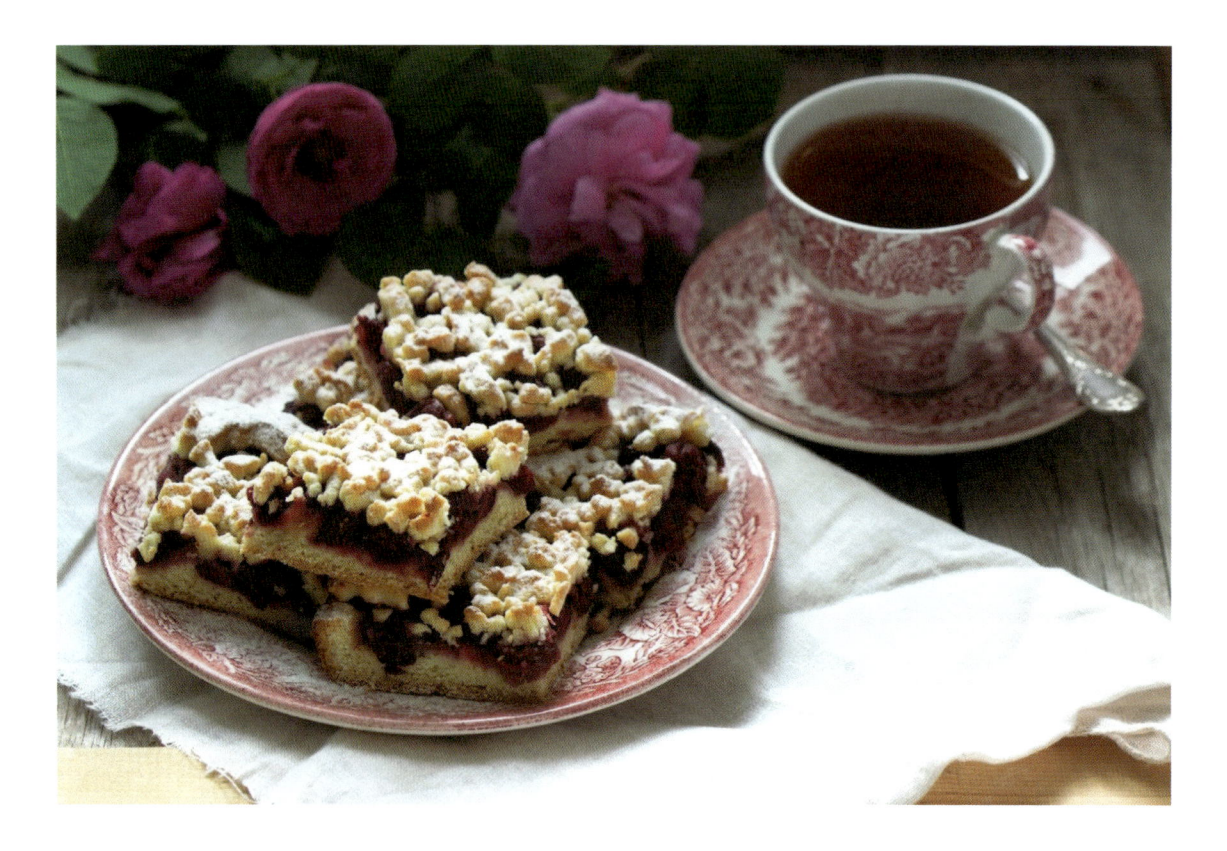

Pecans and almonds are not the only part of this treat; they boost your calcium, too. The bars offer you dietary fiber and heart-healthy fats.

Makes 10 Servings

Cooking + Prep Time: 1/2 hour

Ingredients:

- 3/4 cup of almond butter, creamy
- 1/4 cup of syrup, maple
- 1 tsp. of vanilla extract, pure
- 1/2 tsp. of salt, kosher
- 1 whisked egg white, large
- 2 cups of oats, old-fashioned
- 1/3 cup of pecans
- 1/2 cup of chopped cherries, dried

Instructions:

Preheat the oven to 350F. Line 8" square casserole dish with baking paper.

Combine the almond butter, vanilla, syrup, egg white and salt in large-sized bowl. Whisk, combining well.

Stir in the cherries, oats and pecans. Transfer mixture to 8" dish. Press the mixture into pan firmly.

Bake in 350F oven for 20-22 minutes, till browned lightly. Allow to completely cool. Remove from dish with baking paper. Place on cutting board. Slice & serve.

29 – Fudge-y UC Brownies

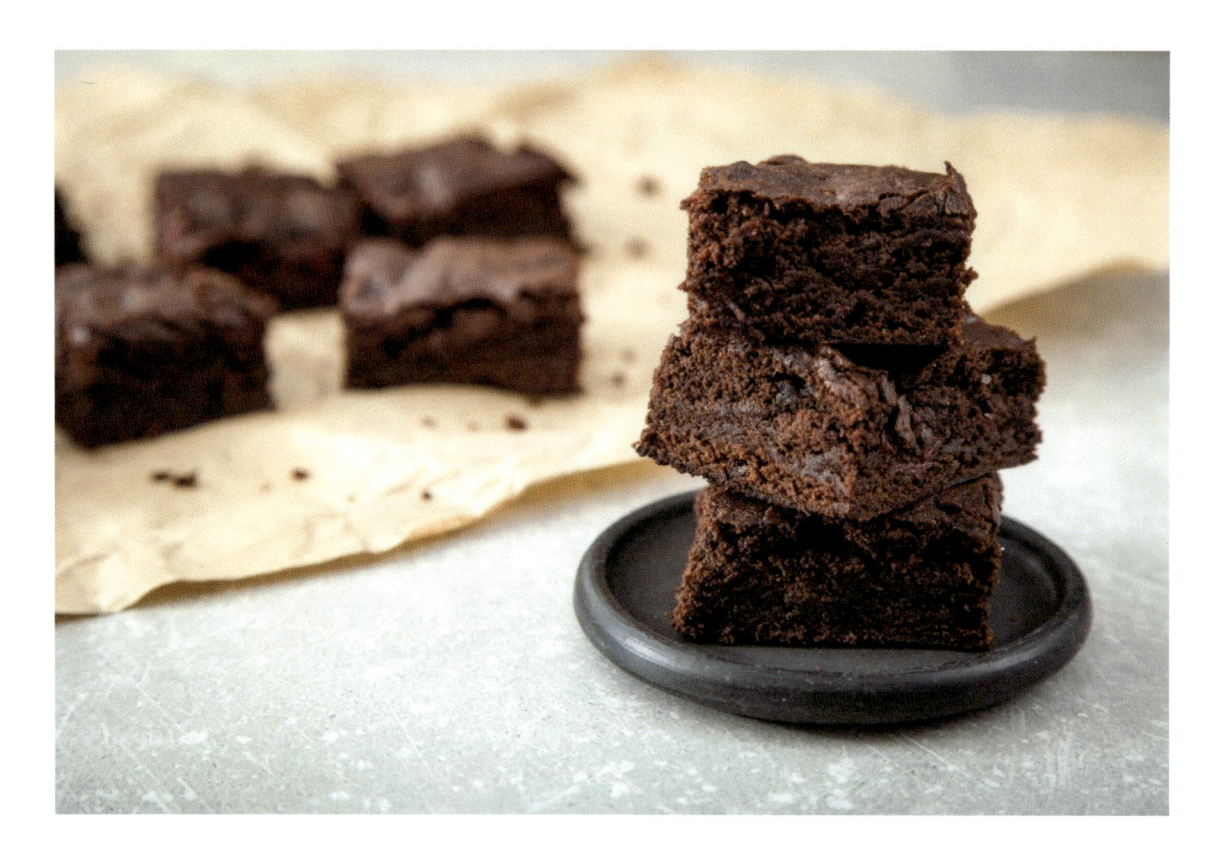

These are healthy, allergen-free brownies that taste like your childhood favorites. The similar taste will surprise you!

Makes Various of Servings

Cooking + Prep Time: 55 minutes

Ingredients:

- 1 cup of oil, coconut
- 1 cup of syrup, maple
- 1 tsp. of vanilla, pure
- 2 eggs, large
- 1/2 cup of flour, tapioca
- 1 cup of cocoa, unsweetened
- 1/4 tsp. of salt, sea
- 1/4 cup of chocolate chips, dairy-free
- 1 tsp. of baking powder

Instructions:

Preheat the oven to 350F. Grease 11-inch x 7-inch baking dish using oil.

Beat oil, syrup, eggs and vanilla in mixing bowl.

In separate mixing bowl, combine cocoa, tapioca, baking powder & salt.

Slowly add dry mixture to wet as you beat them.

Melt chocolate chips using microwave. Add to batter. Stir well. Pour in baking dish. Evenly spread them out.

Bake in 350F oven for 18-20 minutes and serve.

30 – Banana & Strawberry Frosty Dessert

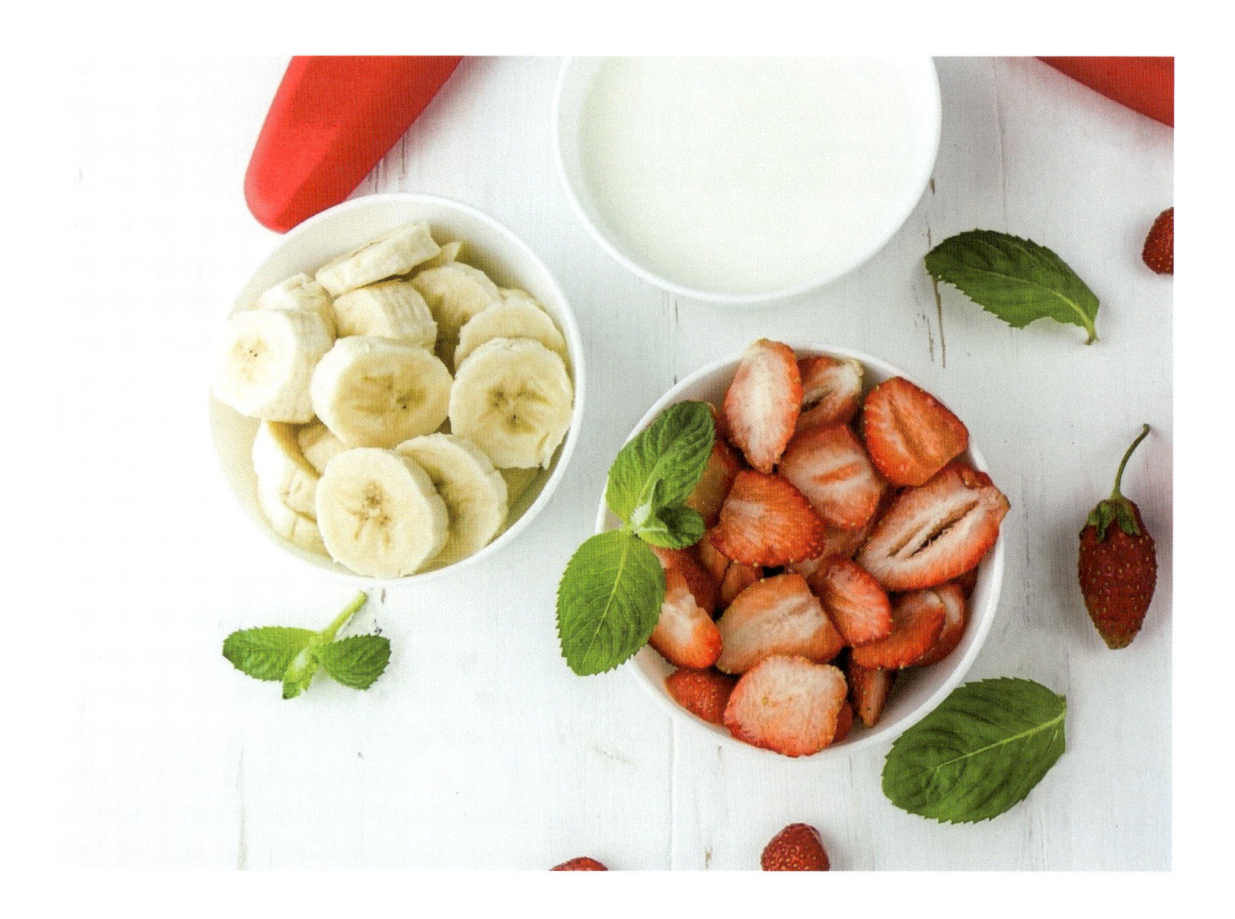

You should still be able to enjoy desserts, even if you have ulcerative colitis. Bananas are among the easiest of fruits to digest, and they help boost potassium.

Makes 2 Servings

Cooking + Prep Time: 15 minutes

Ingredients:

- 1 & 1/2 medium, chopped bananas, frozen
- 1 cup of strawberries, frozen
- 3 tbsp. of milk, vanilla almond, unsweetened

Instructions:

Combine ingredients in food processor. Blend till creamy.

Serve.

Conclusion

This ulcerative colitis cookbook has shown you…

How to use different ingredients to affect unique tastes in many comfort food dishes.

How can you include UC recipes in your home repertoire?

You can…

Make blueberry muffins or sweet potato hash, which you may have heard of before. They are just as tasty as they sound.

Cook soups and stews, which are widely served for UC patients. Find ingredients in meat & produce or frozen food sections of your local grocery stores.

Enjoy making delectable UC seafood dishes, including salmon and trout. Fish is a mainstay in healthy recipes, and there are SO many ways to make it great.

Make dishes using sweet potatoes and pasta for UC friendly meals. There is something about them that makes them more comforting.

Make all kinds of desserts like fudge-y brownies & pineapple cake, which will surely tempt anyone with a sweet tooth.

Enjoy the recipes with your family and friends!

About the Author

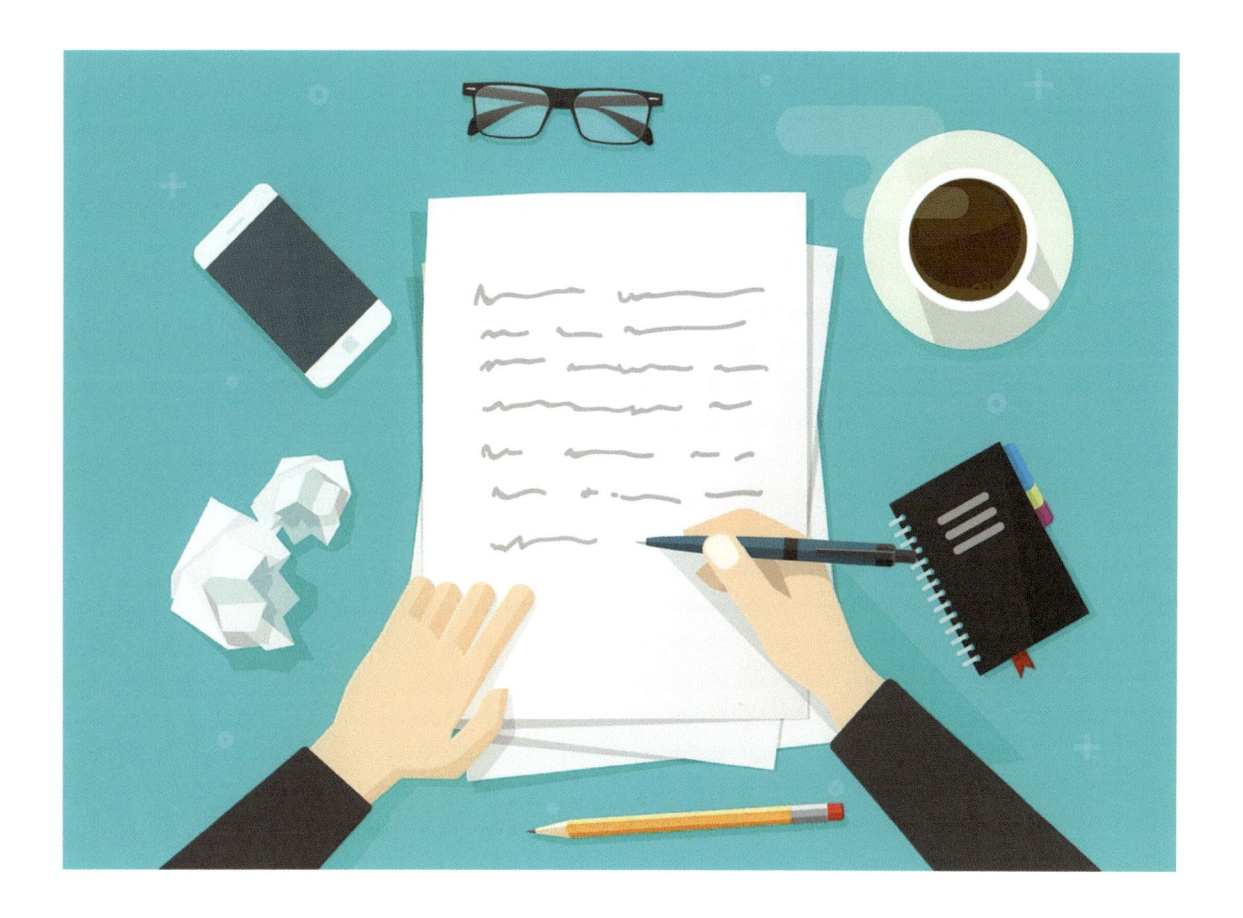

Allie Allen developed her passion for the culinary arts at the tender age of five when she would help her mother cook for their large family of 8. Even back then, her family knew this would be more than a hobby for the young Allie and when she graduated from high school, she applied to cooking school in London. It had always been a dream of the young chef to study with some of Europe's best and she made it happen by attending the Chef Academy of London.

After graduation, Allie decided to bring her skills back to North America and open up her own restaurant. After 10 successful years as head chef and owner, she decided to sell her business and pursue other career avenues. This monumental decision led Allie to her true calling, teaching. She also started to write e-books for her students to study at home for practice. She is now the proud author of several e-books and gives private and semi-private cooking lessons to a range of students at all levels of experience.

Stay tuned for more from this dynamic chef and teacher when she releases more informative e-books on cooking and baking in the near future. Her work is infused with stores and anecdotes you will love!

Author's Afterthoughts

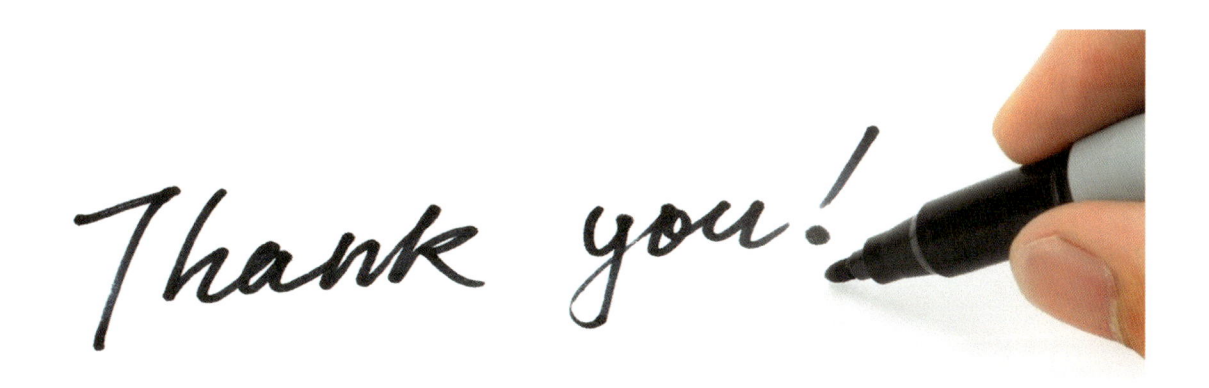

I can't tell you how grateful I am that you decided to read my book. My most heartfelt thanks that you took time out of your life to choose my work and I hope you find benefit within these pages.

There are so many books available today that offer similar content so that makes it even more humbling that you decided to buying mine.

Tell me what you thought! I am eager to hear your opinion and ideas on what you read as are others who are looking for a good book to buy. Leave a review on Amazon.com so others can benefit from your wisdom!

With much thanks,

Allie Allen

Printed in Great Britain
by Amazon